T0073071

Caring for Patients with Depression in Primary Care

David S. Kroll

Caring for Patients with Depression in Primary Care

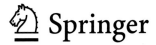 Springer

David S. Kroll
Department of Psychiatry
Brigham and Women's Hospital
Boston, MA, USA

ISBN 978-3-031-08494-2   ISBN 978-3-031-08495-9   (eBook)
https://doi.org/10.1007/978-3-031-08495-9

This Springer imprint is published by the registered company Springer Nature Switzerland AG
The registered company address is: Gewerbestrasse 11, 6330 Cham, Switzerland

For Jeremy.

Acknowledgments

Annie Chakravartti, Kate Gasparrini, Carol Latham, Keona Little, Libby Rodriguez, Laura Shea, Meagan Siciliano, Janice Mahal, Lori Tischler, Bonnie Southworth, Dave Gitlin, Paul Davidson, Martha Byron-Burke, and Lisa Irwin were instrumental in building the psychiatry walk-in clinic, where I gained the clinical experience that I needed to write this book. Helen Higgins, Ali Tapper, Susan Lincoln, Liz Rivera, Madeline Davis, Maria Pires, Nomi Levy-Carrick, Sejal Shah, and Rachael Rosales have made it possible to maintain it. Jane Erb taught me everything I know about depression. Mike Mufson and Marty Kelly taught me everything about disability and the legal system. Thanks as always to David Silbersweig for his unwavering support.

Thanks also to the team at Springer, including Miranda Finch and Josephine Fabiola, for getting this book off the ground.

Chapter 1
Caring for Patients with Depression in Primary Care

How many of you knew you were signing up for this when you decided to go into medicine?

The first (and last) time I asked that question at a CME conference where I was giving a talk about depression for primary care providers, I expected to get a room full of blank stares. I had a whole routine prepared. I assumed that most primary care providers had only come to see treating depression as part of their wheelhouse recently, and only because they had been strongarmed into to by a system that had left the majority of patients without any access to psychiatric specialty care for decades. Everyone was calling primary care the "de facto mental health system," after all [1].

And then about half the audience raised their hands. The other half didn't. For a moment, I was stunned.

But one of the perks about being a psychiatrist is that I have a lot of practice pivoting in conversations. "You see, people's experience with this is highly variable," I finally said, entirely bypassing the joke that I had planned on making, which in retrospect ran a serious risk of falling flat. Maybe nobody noticed that I had missed a beat, and the talk went fine. But I had been put in my place.

The reason that story sticks with me is that I had made the mistake of assuming that primary care providers are a monolith, and this would have been a surefire way to becoming as ineffective as possible in my role as a consulting psychiatrist. *Of course,* the training and experience of primary care providers has been widely variable. This is only natural because their training and experience in treating depression has been *non-systematic*.

I know primary care providers who are completely comfortable managing antipsychotic medications for patients with schizophrenia, or lithium for patients with bipolar disorder. I know others who know all the ins and outs of prescribing antidepressant medications but don't like to go near treating attention deficit-hyperactivity disorder. Some are starting out their careers, or they're in training, or depression wasn't covered enough when they *were* in training, and they just want help with the

D. S. Kroll, *Caring for Patients with Depression in Primary Care*, https://doi.org/10.1007/978-3-031-08495-9_1

basics. Others have completed combined training programs in medicine and psychiatry. Some are working in areas where their patients can usually see a psychiatrist if they want to, and some are working in areas where making a psychiatry referral is like screaming into a void. In other words, different people need different things from a consulting psychiatrist.

I have a unique practice, which is embedded within the Phyllis Jen Center for Primary Care at Brigham and Women's Hospital in Boston, Massachusetts. The practice includes about 150 primary care providers, many of whom are residents training in internal medicine or general medicine, and covers about 17,000 patient lives. We figured out a long time ago that trying to apply a traditional psychiatry practice model didn't work very well for this clinic. Although virtually any medical and social demographic you can think of is represented in the patient population, the patients who were being referred to me were disproportionately those who had significant psychiatric and psychosocial complexity, and many of them had already been kicked out of traditional psychiatry practices due to their being unable to stick to appointments that were usually scheduled months in advance. When I tried to apply the usual set of rules to them, I ended up with nearly a 50% no-show rate and a months-long wait list for new patients [2].

After a few failed attempts of trying to apply traditional strategies to boost attendance in the clinic, one of the social workers came up with the idea that we should just throw scheduling out the window and open up the doors to walk-ins. We tried it, and then things really took off. It turned out that promising same-day (or at least, same-week) access to psychiatric care to any patient who was willing to show up and wait for it did *not* cause the building to explode (as some people seemed to fear it would, based on their extreme anxiety about the idea), and instead it simply opened up more access to very high volume of patients, and disproportionately those who were coming from historically marginalized groups [2, 3]. For a while, we tried to maintain some semblance of control over which patients got referred to the clinic and when, thinking that this might protect us from being overrun by what we imagined to be an unstoppable horde of people who all needed psychiatric care at exactly the same time—like a stampede of Black Friday shoppers at Wal-Mart—but we quickly learned both that it would be impossible to sustain control over the referrals once word got out about the clinic, and that we didn't need to.

By this point, it is a pretty smooth operation. Any patient who receives primary care services in the clinic is invited to come there during walk-in hours and check in for a psychiatry appointment on a first-come, first-served basis. It does not matter how they found out about the clinic, and we don't make them take a survey to tell us about it. They just have to be willing to wait their turn. The way it works is not too different from any other service-oriented business that doesn't rely on appointments or reservations. There are busy days and slow days, but like plenty of barber shops and restaurants, we get by.

The tradeoff for rapid access and high volume is that my clinic is oriented primarily around supporting primary care providers, and not around providing direct longitudinal psychiatric care to patients. I do prescribe, and I see some patients longitudinally, but my chief goal is to help primary care providers get the best outcomes for their patients using either new skills or skills that they already possess but haven't yet been fully honed by experience. It's fairly common, for example, that a primary care provider might start an SSRI and then send the patient for a consult to confirm the right dosing strategy. Or there could be a specific question about side effects, or concern about the risk of underlying bipolar disorder. Sometimes, there are very straightforward questions to be answered, like, "Is it safe to co-prescribe a triptan with an SSRI?" (answer: it's usually fine—see Chap. 4) [4]. Other times, a patient is in a very complicated situation, and the primary care provider doesn't know where to start.

The purpose of this book is similar: to help primary care providers get the best outcomes for their patients with depression, using a combination of new skills and skills that are already there but just need further honing. Unlike the highly heterogenous and variable experience of medical training, however, this book uses a systematic approach to ensure that its content is relentlessly practical and evidence-based.

Chapter 2, **Diagnosing Depression,** starts by addressing the definition of depression and acknowledging that depression is not a single disorder in the way that we commonly speak about it and instead is a highly heterogeneous and multifactorial condition in the real world. This chapter will help you avoid the pitfall of oversimplifying depression when it emerges in your patients and to spot patterns that can be helpful in predicting which patients are more likely to respond to certain treatment plans.

Chapter 3, **Prescribing Antidepressant Medication,** is about the fundamentals of prescribing antidepressant medications, especially the four classes that all share the title of first-line treatment: SSRIs, SNRIs, bupropion, and mirtazapine [5]. In addition to covering the basic skills that clinicians need to prescribe these medications safely and effectively, it teaches you how to choose the right agents for individual patients and then to prescribe them in the most effective, evidence-based way.

Chapter 4, **Managing Risks and Side Effects,** takes a closer look at the risks and side effects that prescribing antidepressant medications entails. It will help you to feel more comfortable balancing the potential risks of any given treatment with its potential benefits, and to discuss these risks more candidly and confidently with patients.

Chapter 5, **Referring to Therapy**, explains how psychotherapy modalities differ from each other and how some might be more or less suitable for individual patients. It also acknowledges the many roadblocks that make many referrals to therapy unsuccessful and offers strategies for overcoming these barriers to get more patients connected.

Chapter 6, **Treatment Resistance and Advanced Therapies**, looks at depression cases that progress beyond the point where first-line treatments apply, and sometimes past the even more distant point where primary care providers ideally should have a supportive role in treatment rather than a leading one. It also teaches you how to spot and manage "pseudoresistance" in depression, a condition in which patients appear to be resistant to treatment but have never actually had an optimized first-line treatment plan.

Chapter 7, **Managing Suicide Risk**, acknowledges that suicide is a possible outcome in patients who have depression as well as in those who do not, and being able to anticipate and manage suicide risk is a skill that all health care providers need to have. Although predicting and preventing suicide 100% of the time is impossible, evidence-based strategies to assess and mitigate suicide risk exist and are readily accessible to primary care clinicians.

Chapter 8, **Managing Conflict**, discusses the inevitable overlap between the patients who have depression and the patients who are more likely to bring conflict into the clinician-patient relationship. It lays out a strategy for resolving disagreements about treatment plans and setting limits around inappropriate or unproductive patient behaviors effectively.

And finally, Chapter 9, **Disability and the Legal System**, anticipates that, because depression is the leading cause of disability in the world, some patients with depression are likely to make requests of their providers that relate to navigating legal systems [6]. This chapter teaches you how to differentiate between your clinical obligations to your patients and a legal agenda that overlaps with but is not always fully aligned with an optimal clinical treatment plan. It also provides guidance on fielding requests to prescribe emotional support animals.

The following chapters are intended to provide a broad and systematic training in treating depression from within a primary care practice. They are also concise. After reading them the first time, you can continue to turn back to them whenever you need to, and you will quickly find the information you need. It will be like having a psychiatry consultant right there in your practice.

References

1. Moise N, Wainberg M, Shah RN. Primary care and mental health: where do we go from here? World J Psychiatry. 2021;11:271–6.
2. Kroll DS, Chakravartti A, Gasparrini K, et al. The walk-in clinic model improves access to psychiatry in primary care. J Psychosom Res. 2016;89:11–5.
3. Kroll DS, Latham C, Mahal J, et al. A successful walk-in psychiatric model for integrated care. J Am Board Fam Med. 2019;32:481–9.
4. Orlova Y, Rizzoli P, Loder E. Association of coprescription of triptan antimigraine drugs and selective serotonin reuptake inhibitor or selective norepinephrine reuptake inhibitor antidepressants with serotonin syndrome. JAMA Neurol. 2018;75:566–72.
5. American Psychiatric Association. Practice guideline for the treatment of patients with major depressive disorder. 3rd ed; 2010.
6. World Health Organization. Depression and other common mental disorders: global health estimates. Geneva: World Health Organization; 2017. License: CC BY-NC-SA 3.0 IGO

Chapter 2
Diagnosing Depression

The word "depression" can conjure up a lot of dread. Often, if I ask a patient whether they feel depressed, they will reply with something along the lines of, "I don't know, doctor—you tell me!" Of course, how could I possibly know how anyone else is feeling? But they—and many, many others—have mistakenly conflated this highly stigmatized emotional state with a clinical diagnosis.

Depressed mood—like pain, swelling, weakness, or any other unpleasant feeling—is a highly common and nonspecific experience that requires context to understand. Not everyone who feels depressed at any point in time has major depressive disorder just like not everyone who has a headache has a migraine disorder. Even a diagnosis of major depressive disorder can mean different things for different people. Consider the following three patients:

1. *Anna is a 28-year-old woman with a significant trauma history dating back to childhood. She first attempted suicide when she was 11 years old and was hospitalized for recurrent suicidal ideation and suicide attempts at least six times before the age of 16. After she was finally emancipated from her abusive childhood home, her depression significantly improved (although never fully remitted) and remained in a state of relative stability until age 22, when her first child was born to man who intermittently abused her. She finally extracted herself and her daughter from this relationship when she was 25 and has since been living in a family shelter. She has not worked in 7 years and now collects disability income as a result of her depressive disorder. She endorses depressed mood on a daily basis, but she has not thought about suicide since her daughter was born. She is not sleeping well as a result of her shelter environment not being conducive to this, but she feels excessively tired and unable to concentrate during the day. She has a history of trauma-related nightmares and previously met diagnostic criteria for PTSD, but these symptoms have abated and now only rarely bother her. She describes herself as an emotional eater, and she has a relatively non-nutritious diet. As a result, her BMI has steadily risen over the years to a*

D. S. Kroll, *Caring for Patients with Depression in Primary Care*, https://doi.org/10.1007/978-3-031-08495-9_2

recent peak of 39. She has tried multiple antidepressant and mood-stabilizing medications over the years—including sertraline, escitalopram, bupropion, trazodone, venlafaxine, lamotrigine, and lurasidone—but has had only a modest benefit from these.

2. *Sheila is a 36-year-old woman whose second lifetime major depressive episode began after the birth of her second child. Her first episode had seemed to occur spontaneously when she was 29, and it fully remitted after 6 months of treatment on citalopram. Approximately 1 month after her second child was born, however, she began to feel like she had during her first episode—anxious, irritable, and depressed. She was also sleeping poorly—so was her baby—her energy was terrible during the day, and she couldn't concentrate. The idea of suicide briefly crossed her mind, although she never considered these thoughts seriously or developed a suicide plan. However, she felt excessively guilty about the fact that suicidal thoughts had even occurred to her and about what she perceived to be a lack of enthusiasm for mothering. You restart citalopram, and approximately 3 months later, her symptoms significantly improve. After another 3 months, she feels totally back to her baseline, and she successfully discontinues her medication.*

3. *Lawrence is a 72-year-old man who lost his wife 1 year ago to a sudden infectious illness. He had no prior psychiatric history, but since becoming widowed, he has felt like a "different person." He no longer enjoys any of the hobbies he and his wife used to engage in, and he spends most of his time during the day sleeping or watching television. He has lost interest in socializing and rarely goes out. He no longer bathes regularly, and he sometimes forgets to eat. He has lost about 30 lbs, although he had been overweight before. He has also started missing his appointments with you, which he never previously did, and you have had to involve a visiting nurse in his care in order to ensure that he takes his other medications. According to the visiting nurse, he is accepting of her care, but his apartment is filthy.*

It is remarkable that all of three of these patients share the exact same clinical diagnosis: major depressive disorder, or MDD. The diagnostic criteria for MDD (Fig. 2.1) allow for an enormous degree of heterogeneity in how affected patients may present—arguably more so than in most other recognized diseases. This would imply, of course, that MDD is expected to present in a wide variety of different ways (like syphilis), but also that any patient who meets the diagnostic criteria by any of its permutations has the same disease as everyone else and, by extension, should have the same prognosis and the same expectation of responding to the same treatments [1].

This premise can be difficult to accept. To qualify for a diagnosis of MDD, it makes no difference at all if a patient has insomnia or hypersomnia, a loss of appetite or an excessive appetite, psychomotor slowing or agitation. It makes no more difference if the disorder lasts for 2 months or 20 years; if it began in childhood,

At least 5 of the following, including either criterion 1 or 2, must be present for at least 2 weeks:

1. Depressed or irritable mood for most of the day, almost every day
2. A loss of interest or pleasure in almost activities
3. Significant increase or decrease in appetite or weight
4. Insomnia or hypersomnia
5. Psychomotor agitation or retardation
6. Fatigue or loss of energy
7. Feelings of worthlessness or guilt
8. Impaired concentration or indecisiveness
9. Recurrent thoughts of death or suicide, or suicidal behavior

In addition, the symptoms must cause clinically significant distress or impairment and cannot be attributable to a substance or general medical condition.

Fig. 2.1 Summary of diagnostic criteria for Major Depressive Disorder [2]

adulthood, or late life; if it emerged spontaneously or as a reaction to trauma or stress; or even if it is responsive to treatment. Depression simply equals MDD if the right criteria occur along with it, which some critics have argued are overly broad. Some authors have in fact pointed out that if all the possible symptoms and symptom variations that are listed in the DSM-5 are considered, over 16,000 different symptom profiles for MDD are possible [1]!

This unifying approach to diagnosing MDD, which relies heavily on the patient's phenotypic presentation at a specific moment in time, naturally runs the risk of conflating what could be a number of different disease processes. It also implies that the timing and nature of the condition's onset and its longitudinal course are not as diagnostically important. With some exceptions, we still do not know how relevant most of these factors are in differentiating between types and subtypes of major depression, if they are truly distinct entities at all. They may have serious implications for treatment, or they may not.

What we do know is that depression is complicated. As we go through the nuances of diagnosing depression correctly—to the extent that the available evidence makes this possible—it is important to always keep in mind that depression is **heterogeneous** and **multifactorial**. Even in spite of all the benefits that an algorithmic approach to treatment can bring to your practice (which I do not intend to undermine here—see Chap. 3), there really cannot be a one-size-fits-all solution to diagnosing or treating depression because it is not a single, straightforward thing.

Ignoring life experiences and other environmental factors for a moment, there are multiple biochemical processes that have been shown to have a role in the development of depressive disorders, either independently or in relation to each other, at least some of the time. These include primary neurological functions, neurotransmitter activity, hormonal activity, and inflammation. Their mechanisms are more omplicated than we need to get into for the purposes of this chapter, but here is a brief summary:

The term "neuroplasticity" refers to the nervous system's ability to change and adapt to its internal and external environments, and several theories about depression intersect at this concept. In this framework, depression may be the result of impaired neuroplasticity, and the brains of patients with depression have fewer synaptic connections and show signs of neuronal atrophy [3]. These changes in turn impair functioning in multiple bodily systems and lead to decreased cognitive flexibility, perhaps also making it more difficult to challenge persistent negative thoughts and biases [3]. Serotonin modulates neuronal plasticity [4], and this role may partly explain why serotonergic medications can be effective in treating depression. However, serotonin has many functions that likely relate to mood regulation, and many other factors also affect plasticity, including other neurotransmitters, genetics, intracellular events, and stress [3].

At the same time, some patients with depression have structural changes in the brain that can be observed on MRI, including decreased volume in the hippocampus and prefrontal cortex [3]. Neurodegenerative and cerebrovascular illnesses that disrupt certain brain areas or circuits can similarly result in depression [5].

Systemic hormonal changes or deficiencies are also implicated. Excess activity of the hypothalamic-pituitary-adrenal (HPA) axis has been linked to several types of depression, and hypercortisolemia is a highly common finding in depressed patients [4, 6]. The symptoms of hypothyroidism and male hypogonadism can include depression [7, 8], and some patterns of depression occur in women exclusively during times of hormonal flux (e.g., perimenstrual depression and peripartum depression) [8]. Depression has also been associated with lower levels of vitamin D, folic acid, and vitamin B12, supporting a possible link between diet and depression, although the nature and strength of this link is not well understood [9–12].

Finally, injecting a Salmonella endotoxin intravenously into healthy test subjects produces a transient state of depression [13]. There is a strong association between higher levels of inflammatory cytokines (particularly interleukin-6, IL-6, and tumor necrosis factor-α, TNF-α) and depression, and anti-inflammatory medications can reduce depression symptoms in some cases [14–16]. The reverse is also true: treatment with antidepressant medications can reduce inflammatory cytokines [17, 18]. These findings have led to the development of an inflammatory hypothesis for depression, which maintains that systemic inflammation underlies some depressive disorders, possibly by affecting neuroplasticity [4].

Any or all of these processes may be more or less relevant to the case of an individual patient. The purpose of describing them here is not to give you the tools you would need to apply a true precision medicine approach to treating depression—this would be great, but the field is simply not there yet—but rather to illustrate how heterogeneous and multifactorial depression is in real patients. Making a diagnosis—which remains a necessary part of providing care—almost always means oversimplifying the problem.

That said, the established diagnoses are a good place to start. MDD may be particularly tricky because the diagnostic criteria are so flexible and broad, but even within this diagnosis there are recurring patterns that have been studied as distinct clinical entities and can inform initial treatment planning. Some of these entities (melancholic features, atypical features, seasonal pattern, etc.) are acknowledged within the DSM-5 and can be indicated in the diagnosis by the use of modifiers. Where there is a lack of a clear distinction between some different types of depression in current diagnostic classification schemes, keep in mind that this is not a result of ignorance or laziness on behalf of the experts who wrote the manuals. Instead, the data simply are not clear enough to inform us on where exactly to draw the lines between one type or another. Classic melancholic symptoms (see below) also correlate with symptom severity, further confounding this difficulty [19].

Melancholic depression, or melancholia, may be the most easily recognizable form of MDD and appears to be the predominant pattern in 20–30% of all cases [19–22]. Patients with melancholic depression present in adulthood with severe depression and anhedonia, and they exhibit the most classic neurovegetative changes: early morning awakening, a loss of appetite, and psychomotor retardation [20, 23, 24]. Their depressed mood also tends to be more severe in the morning, and it improves throughout the day [23]. Distinct cognitive changes, including impairments in memory, attention, executive functioning, and psychomotor changes can be found on neuropsychological testing, and these are more pronounced than in other subtypes of MDD [20].

Melancholic depression is often referred to as an "endogenous" or "autonomous" depression because it is associated with a relative unresponsiveness to environmental factors [21, 25]. While stress can precede the onset of this condition, it is less likely than some other types of depression to occur in direct response to a severe stressful life event [26]. It is similarly less likely to improve with non-medical treatment approaches, including psychotherapy and placebos [27, 28]. Instead, treatment of melancholic depression classically requires the use of a medication or other somatic treatment [21, 24, 28].

The term "**atypical depression**" can be used to refer to virtually any kind of MDD that is not melancholic, although it is most commonly used to describe a specific pattern characterized by hypersomnia, increased appetite, and interpersonal rejection sensitivity. Symptoms are characteristically more severe in the evening [22]. An atypical pattern of depression is associated with an early age of onset, female sex, a stronger family history (of both atypical depression and bipolar disorder), and co-morbid dysthymia, personality disorders, low self-esteem, and substance use [20, 22, 23]. Mood reactivity can be a prominent feature, and patients are more likely to develop symptoms following severe stressful life events [20, 26]. Psychotherapy has a more critical role in this type of depression, although it also responds especially well to monoamine oxidase inhibitors (MAOIs) [29].

Peripartum depression (a.k.a., MDD with peripartum onset) is defined as an episode of major depressive disorder that has its onset during pregnancy or within the first 4 weeks postpartum. It is estimated to affect up to 20% of women in the peripartum period, and the true prevalence may be even higher than this [30, 31]. It is etiologically linked to other types of MDD as well as to the unique psychosocial stressors that pregnant women and new mothers are burdened with in most societies

[9]. However, an additional role for hormonal shifts related to reproductive functions and the HPA axis has also been postulated [30]. Brexanolone, an intravenous preparation of allopregnanalone, is uniquely effective for rapidly reversing the symptoms of postpartum depression, supporting this hypothesis [31].

Dysthymia (a.k.a., persistent depressive disorder) (Fig. 2.2) is a chronic depressive condition marked by persistent mild-to-moderate depression and often has its onset in childhood. This diagnosis is historically associated with the concept of neuroticism and a depressive personality style, but in practice it is also strongly associated with MDD and a positive response to antidepressant medications [32]. Neurovegetative symptoms are less common [23]. Dysthymia is commonly misdiagnosed as MDD in practice and research, but these two conditions can also co-occur in the same patient [23, 32].

It should also be noted that the DSM-5 characterizes dysthymia as a consolidation of the DSM-IV diagnosis of dysthymic disorder with chronic MDD, and cases of prolonged major depressive episodes (beyond 2 years) could be given diagnoses of both MDD and dysthymic disorder [2].

An **adjustment disorder** (Fig. 2.3) is a psychological response to stressful life events or losses that is beyond what would ordinarily be expected. One could reasonably point out that this is almost by definition a murky concept. Who is to say

---

1. Depressed mood for most of the day, more often than not, for at least 2 years
2. At least 2 of the following: high or low appetite, insomnia or hypersomnia, low
   energy, low self-esteem, impaired concentration or indecisiveness, feelings of hopelessness.
3. No periods of symptom remission lasting longer than 2 months
4. If criteria for MDD have been met continuously for a full 2 years, this also qualifies for
   dysthymia, but not if they have only been present for part of this period.
5. No history of mania, hypomania, or cyclothymia
6. Symptoms are not better explained by a psychotic disorder, substance or medication use,
   or another medical condition
7. Symptoms cause clinically significant distress or impairment

Fig. 2.2 Summary of diagnostic criteria for Persistent Depressive Disorder [2]

---

1. Emotional or behavioral symptoms develop within 3 months of the onset of an
   identifiable stressor
2. Distress is out of proportion to what would be expected in the context, taking cultural factors
   into account—or there is significant functional impairment
3. Symptoms do not represent normal bereavement or meet criteria for another disorder
   and do not represent an exacerbation of a pre-existing disorder
4. Symptoms remit within 6 months of the stressor or its consequences resolving

Fig. 2.3 Summary of diagnostic criteria for Adjustment Disorder [2]

what constitutes an excessive response to stress? And yet, this is among the most common diagnoses given to patients by behavioral health specialists [33].

Commonly referred to as a "situational" depression, an adjustment disorder emerges as a direct response to a stressful or distressing event or situation. It should also resolve spontaneously over time or with the removal of the stress that triggered it. However, symptoms can be prolonged in cases where the stressful situation cannot be resolved. The optimal role of treatment in adjustment disorders remains unclear, in part because adjustment disorders are temporary and in part because the quality of research into this condition is poor [34]. However, both medication and psychotherapy can be helpful in some cases [35].

Bipolar disorder is theoretically identifiable by the presence of manic or hypomanic episodes, but many patients with bipolar disorder present primarily, or even exclusively, with recurrent depression. It can therefore be very difficult to distinguish from MDD, particularly at a single moment in time and early in the course of the disorder, before any manic or hypomanic symptoms have had a chance to emerge. However, some characteristic features may lead you to consider this diagnosis.

It is a life-long condition. Its onset usually occurs in late adolescence or early adulthood, and it follows a cyclic course with (usually) distinct episodes [36, 37]. Depressive episodes are more likely to include atypical features (as in atypical depression) or psychotic features [23, 37], and affected patients are also more likely to have a history of impulsivity, substance abuse, and personality disorders even if a clear history of manic episodes cannot be identified [37]. It is also strongly impacted by genetic factors, and a family history of bipolar disorder should be considered a clue to this diagnosis [38].

Although the majority of patients with bipolar disorder are treated with conventional antidepressant medications, their use in this condition is controversial at best [39]. While antidepressants can lead to improved depression symptoms in the short-term, they do not improve long-term outcomes, and instead they can increase the frequency of depressive episodes or trigger a manic episode [39]. Therefore, they are generally not recommended in bipolar disorder. Patients who have been diagnosed with bipolar disorder or have a symptom pattern that is strongly suggestive of bipolar disorder should be prioritized for a referral to psychiatry for management, if this resource is available.

Cyclothymia is (probably) a variant of bipolar disorder that follows a milder course. Patients with cyclothymia can develop periodic mild to moderate depression symptoms (classically with atypical features) and hypomanic phases that are usually brief in duration and are more likely to involve prominent irritability rather than euphoria or heightened productivity [40]. They are also prone to intense mood swings, and cyclothymia can be difficult to differentiate from a personality disorder [40]. Optimal treatment strategies are not well-established, but a common approach is to treat this similarly to bipolar disorder [40].

Seasonal affective disorder (SAD) is thought to be etiologically related to the decrease in natural light availability during the fall and winter months at latitudes where this is relevant [41]. Depression typically follows an annual pattern in which it emerges in the fall and resolves in the spring or summer, and some patients develop hypomania in the summer [23, 41]. Although antidepressant medication and psychotherapy can both be helpful, light therapy is the mainstay of treatment and should be discussed with patients who present with seasonal depression [41, 42]. Patients should be advised to purchase their light therapy device from a reliable source, and their device should be designed specifically for the treatment of SAD (i.e., it should not advertise that it simply elevates the mood, as this can reflect a misleading marketing strategy for an inferior product). For light therapy to be optimally effective, the patient should sit between 12–18 inches from their device, at an angle from their vision, for approximately 30 minutes every morning from early-to-mid autumn until spring [41]. Alternatively, traveling to a more temperate latitude can also help for those who have the resources and flexibility to do so.

Premenstrual dysphoric disorder (PMDD) is a cyclical mood disorder that occurs in anatomically female patients beginning in the week before the start of menses and remitting before the end of menses. Although depression is a common symptom of PMDD, irritability and mood instability are the more prominent symptoms [43]. Its etiology is believed to be hormonally based, but its pathophysiology is not yet well understood [44]. Although the symptoms are predictable and short-lived, they can be seriously impairing or distressing in some patients. It should also be noted that not all patients who experience mood changes perimenstrually qualify for a diagnosis of PMDD, and these milder symptoms are commonly referred to as premenstrual syndrome, or PMS, although PMS is not considered to be a psychiatric disorder [43].

SSRIs are the mainstay of treatment for PMDD. However, unlike in other mood disorders, SSRIs can be effective for PMDD even if they are dosed intermittently. Typically, they are prescribed beginning at the time of ovulation, or 14 days prior to the start of menses every month [43, 44]. Some regimens involve starting the medication only after the onset of symptoms, but this strategy is less effective [44]. Continuous contraception is also sometimes used to treat PMDD, but the evidence supporting its efficacy is less robust [43, 44].

Personality disorders commonly cause both chronic and episodic mood changes and also commonly co-occur with other depressive disorders. Patients with personality disorders have life-long mood disturbances that are often characterized primarily by mood instability, anger, and extreme emotional sensitivity as opposed to persistent or pervasive depression and anhedonia, and they do not necessarily exhibit neurovegetative symptoms [45]. However, they might still meet diagnostic criteria for another mood disorder at specific points in time—because most mood disorders are diagnosed based on symptoms that occur at a particular point in time rather than their longitudinal course, this is perhaps an inevitable pitfall [45]. Distinguishing between the symptoms of a personality disorder and the other diagnoses that they may qualify for at one time or another (correctly or incorrectly) can therefore be difficult.

In general, the depression that occurs in the context of personality disorders is more difficult to treat and is more likely to be associated with a worse outcome [46,

47]. An interdisciplinary team approach is generally recommended. It is also important to recognize that the maladaptive emotional and behavioral responses that are the hallmark of these disorders can also occur in patients who do not necessarily meet criteria for a personality disorder [46]. Many people can present with narcissistic or borderline traits, for example, to a milder degree or only in certain situations without having the full spectrum of problems that a true personality disorder entails. However, these traits can still be impairing at times and can get in the way of treatment [47].

The concept of a **mood disorder secondary to a general medical condition** implies that the mood symptoms the affected patient is experiencing are driven entirely by an underlying medical process and that reversing the medical condition should rapidly resolve them. A common example is hypothyroidism: a hypothyroid state can produce depressed mood and psychomotor slowing, and this process has little to do with how we otherwise understand depression. This form of depression is not treated with antidepressants or psychotherapy and instead requires correcting the thyroid hormone deficit. However, in practice, this is rarely so simple.

Medical conditions do not occur in a vacuum, so to speak. Having a chronic medical condition in particular often means living with symptoms, disruptions to daily life, and sometimes disability and/or disfigurement—all of which can be unpleasant and stressful and thus can activate more conventional psychological processes that contribute to a depressed mood state. Meanwhile, any inflammation or activation of the HPA axis that occurs as a direct result of the underlying medical condition might similarly overlap with other physiologic processes that may be associated with a purely "neuropsychiatric" depression (or may even represent a different form of depression secondary to a general medical condition).

In other words, everything intersects with everything else. A good example to illustrate how this works in the real world is neuropsychiatric lupus. Systemic lupus erythematosus (SLE) is thought to possibly exert direct neuropsychiatric effects through multiple mechanisms, including cerebrovascular dysfunction, antibody activity against N-methyl-D-aspartate (NMDA) receptors, disruption of the blood-brain barrier, and inflammation [48–51]. At the same time, patients with SLE suffer from chronic pain, fatigue, disrupted sleep, a lower quality of life, and at times a disfigured appearance (or at least a perception of one) [52, 53]. Thus, a combination of systemic, neuropsychiatric, and psychological factors converges to produce an altered mood state in a patient for whom optimal treatment would likely be multi-modal.

The idea behind a **substance-induced mood disorder** is similar: certain substances (including prescribed medications) can directly produce a depressed phenotype outside of its direct intoxication or withdrawal effects. Antihypertensive agents are a commonly cited example of a type of substance that can be associated with a secondary depression, although this association may not even truly exist [54]. As in depressive disorders that are secondary to a general medical condition, substance-induced mood disorders are usually multifactorial in real clinical practice.

Chemical substances—including those that are commonly used nonmedically— can impact the course of depression in a variety of ways. Alcohol in particular has a complex and bidirectional relationship with depression, and when alcohol use disorders and depression occur together, their combination is usually associated with an increased disease severity and worse outcomes [55, 56]. Long-term opioid use, even when it is prescribed, can similarly increase the risk of developing more severe and treatment-refractory depression [57]. Substance use disorders and personality disorders also commonly occur together, further confounding the diagnosis [58]. However, if the depression is purely substance-induced, it should resolve within weeks of discontinuing the substance [56]. If it does not, to describe the depression as a dual diagnosis condition (i.e., comorbid depressive and substance use disorders) would be more accurate.

This list is not exhaustive. Other depressive states have been described, and undoubtedly, some patterns that have not yet been recognized will be described in the future. However, the take-home point is that depression is a highly heterogenous and multifactorial condition. Some types are driven chiefly by physiologic processes and are best treated medically, and others are more closely related to psychological and behavioral patterns that may respond better to psychological or behavioral treatments. Most fall somewhere in between these two extremes, and often there is a role for multiple kinds of treatment.

References

1. Fried EI, Nesse RM. Depression is not a consistent syndrome: an investigation of unique symptom patterns in the STAR*d study. J Affect Disord. 2015;172:96–102.
2. American Psychiatric Association. Diagnostic and statistical manual of mental disorders (DSM-5). 5th ed. Arlington, Virginia: American Psychiatric Association; 2013.
3. Price RB, Duman R. Neuroplasticity in cognitive and psychological mechanisms of depression: an integrative model. Mol Psychiatry. 2020;25:530–43.
4. Kraus C, Castrén E, Kasper S, Lanzenberger R. Serotonin and neuroplasticity—links between molecular, functional and structural pathophysiology in depress. Neurosci Biobehav Rev. 2017;77:317–26.
5. Bour A, Rasquin S, Aben I, et al. A one-year follow-up study into the course of depression after stroke. J Nutr Health Aging. 2010;14:488–93.
6. Keller J, Gomez R, Williams G, et al. HPA axis in major depression: cortisol, clinical symptomatology and genetic variation predict cognition. Mol Psychiatry. 2017;22:527–36.
7. Siegmann E, Müller HHO, Luecke C, et al. Association of depression and anxiety disorders with autoimmune thyroiditis: a systematic review and meta-analysis. JAMA Psychiat. 2018;75:577–84.
8. McHenry J, Carrier N, Hull E, Kabbaj M. Sex differences in anxiety and depression: role of testosterone. Front Neuroendocrinol. 2014;42:57.
9. Parker BG, Brotchie H, Graham RK. Vitamin D and depression. J Affect Disord. 2017;208:56–61.
10. Bender A, Hagan KE, Kingston N. The association of folate and depression: a meta-analysis. J Psychiatr Res. 2017;95:9–18.
11. Khosravi M, Sotoudeh G, Amini M, et al. The relationship between dietary patterns and depression mediated by serum levels of folate at vitamin B12. BMC Psychiatry. 2020;20:63.
12. Molendijk M, Molero P, Sánchez-Pedreño FO, et al. Diet quality and depression risk: a systematic review and dose-response meta-analysis of prospective studies. J Affect Disord. 2018;226:346–54.

13. Reichenberg A, Yirmiya R, Schuld R, et al. Cytokine-associated emotional and cognitive disturbances in humans. Arch Gen Psychiatry. 2001;58:445–52.
14. Dowlati Y, Hermann N, Swardfager W, et al. A meta-analysis of cytokines in major depression. Biol Psychiatry. 2010;67:446–57.
15. Krishnan R, Cella D, Leonard C, et al. Effects of etanercept therapy on fatigue and symptoms of depression in subjects treated for moderate to severe plaque psoriasis for up to 96 weeks. Br J Dermatol. 2007;157:1275–7.
16. Abbasi S, Hosseini F, Modabbernia A, et al. Effect of celecoxib add-on treatment on symptoms and serum IL-6 concentrations in patients with major depressive disorder: randomized double-blind placebo-controlled study. J Affect Disord. 2012;141:308–14.
17. Hannestad J, DellaGiola N, Block M. The effect of antidepressant medication treatment on serum levels of inflammatory cytokines: a meta-analysis. Neuropsychopharmacology. 2011;36:2452–9.
18. Liu JJ, Wei YB, Strawbridge R, et al. Peripheral cytokine levels and response to antidepressant treatment in depression: a systematic review and meta-analysis. Mol Psychiatry. 2020;25:339–50.
19. Tondo L, Vázquez GH, Baldessarini RJ. Melancholic versus nonmelancholic major depression compared. J Affect Disord. 2020;266:760–5.
20. Bosaipo NB, Foss MP, Young AH, Juruena MF. Neuropsychological changes in melancholic and atypical depression: a systematic review. Neurosci Biobehav Rev. 2017;73:309–25.
21. Day CVA, Williams LM. Finding a biosignature for melancholic depression. Expert Rev Neurother. 2012;12:835–47.
22. Juruena MF, Cleare AJ. Overlap between atypical depression, seasonal affective disorder and chronic fatigue syndrome. Rev Bras Psiquiatr. 2007;29:S19–26.
23. Benazzi F. Various forms of depression. Dialogues Clin Neurosci. 2006;8:151–61.
24. Parker G, Tavella G, Hadzi-Pavlovic D. Identifying and differentiating melancholic depression in a non-clinical sample. J Affect Disord. 2019;243:194–200.
25. Ghaemi SN, Vohringer PA. The heterogeneity of depression: an old debate renewed. Acta Psychiatr Scand. 2011;124:497.
26. Harkness KL, Monroe SM. Severe melancholic depression is more vulnerable than non-melancholic depression to minor precipitating life events. J Affect Disord. 2006;91:257–63.
27. Mizushima J, Sakurai H, Mizuno Y, et al. Melancholic and reactive depression: a reappraisal of old categories. BMC Psychiatry. 2013;13:311.
28. Peselow ED, Sanfilipo MP, Difiglia C, Fieve RR. Melancholic/endogenous depression and response to somatic treatment and placebo. Am J Psychiatry. 1992;149:1324–34.
29. Parker G, Roy K, Mitchell P, et al. Atypical depression: a reappraisal. Am J Psychiatry. 2002;159:1470–9.
30. Payne JL, Maguire J. Pathophysiological mechanisms implicated in postpartum depression. Front Neuroendocrinol. 2019;52:165–80.
31. Zheng W, Cai D, Zheng W, et al. Brexanolone for postpartum depression: a meta-analysis of randomized controlled studies. Psychiatry Res. 2019;279:83–9.
32. Schramm E, Klein DN, Elsaesser M, et al. Review of dysthymia and persistent depressive disorder: history, correlates, and clinical implications. Lancet Psychiatry. 2002;7:801–12.
33. Bachem R, Casey P. Adjustment disorder: a diagnosis whose time has come. J Affect Disord. 2018;227:243–53.
34. O'Donnell ML, Metcalf O, Watson L, et al. A systematic review of psychological and pharmacological treatments for adjustment disorder in adults. J Trauma Stress. 2018;31:321–31.
35. Casey P. Adjustment disorder: epidemiology, diagnosis and treatment. CNS Drugs. 2009;23:927–38.
36. McIntyre RS, Calabrese JR. Bipolar depression: the clinical characteristics and unmet needs of a complex disorder. Curr Med Res Opin. 2019;35:1993–2005.
37. Aiken CB, Weisler RH, Sachs GS. The bipolarity index: a clinician-rated measure of diagnostic confidence. J Affect Disord. 2015;177:59–64.
38. Craddock N, Sklar P. Genetics of bipolar disorder. Lancet. 2013;381:1654–62.

39. Ghaemi SN. Why antidepressants are not antidepressants: STEP-BD, STAR*D, and the return of neurotic depression. Bipolar Disord. 2008;10:957–68.
40. Perugi G, Hantouche E, Vannucchi G, Pinto O. Cyclothymia reloaded: a reappraisal of the most misconceived affective disorder. J Affect Disord. 2015;183:119–33.
41. Kurlansik SL, Ibay AD. Seasonal affective disorder. Am Fam Physician. 2012;86:1037–41.
42. Meyerhoff J, Young MA, Rohan KJ. Patterns of depressive symptom remission during the treatment of seasonal affective disorder with cognitive-behavioral therapy or light therapy. Depress Anxiety. 2018;35:457–67.
43. Hantsoo L, Epperson CN. Premenstrual dysphoric disorder: epidemiology and treatment. Curr Psychiatry Rep. 2015;17:87.
44. Carlini SV, Deligiannidis KM. Evidence-based treatment of premenstrual dysphoric disorder: a concise review. J Clin Psychiatry. 2020;81:19ac13071.
45. Fjermestad-Noll J, Ronningstam E, Bach B, et al. Characterological depression in patients with narcissistic personality disorder. Nord J Psychiatry. 2019;73:539–45.
46. Newton-Howes G, Tyrer P, Johnson T. Personality disorder and the outcome of depression: meta-analysis of published studies. Br J Psychiatry. 2006;188:13–20.
47. Luca M, Luca A, Calandra C. Borderline personality disorder and depression: an update. Psychiatry Q. 2012;83:281–92.
48. Rhiannon JJ. Systemic lupus erythematosus involving the nervous system: presentation, pathogenesis, and management. Clin Rev Allergy Immunol. 2008;34:356–60.
49. Omdal R, Brokstad K, Waterloo K, Koldingsnes W, Jonsson R, Mellgren SI. Neuropsychiatric disturbances in SLE are associated with antibodies against NMDA receptors. Eur J Neurol. 2005;12:392–298.
50. Abbot NJ, Mendonca LLF, Dolman DEM. The blood-brain barrier in systemic lupus erythematosus. Lupus. 2003;12:908–15.
51. Fragoso-Loyo H, Richaud-Patin Y, Orozco-Narvaez A, et al. Interleukin-6 and chemokines in the neuropsychiatric manifestations of systemic lupus erythematosus. Arthritis Rheum. 2007;56(4):1242–50.
52. Iverson GL. Screening for depression in systemic lupus erythematosus with the British Columbia major depression inventory. Psychol Rep. 2002;90:1091–6.
53. Monaghan SM, Sharpe L, Denton F, Levy J, Schrieber L, Sensky T. Relationship between appearance and psychological distress in rheumatic diseases. Arthritis Rheum. 2007;57(2):303–9.
54. Kessing LV, Rytgaard HC, Ekstrøm CT, et al. Antihypertensive drugs and risk of depression: a nationwide population-based study. Hypertension. 2020;76:1263–79.
55. Pavkovic B, Zaric M, Markovic M, et al. Double screening for dual disorder, alcoholism and depression. Psychiatry Res. 2018;270:483–9.
56. McHugh RK, Weiss RD. Alcohol use disorder and depressive disorders. Alcohol Res. 2019;40:arcr.v40.1.01.
57. Sullivan MD. Depression effects on long-term prescription opioid use, abuse, and addiction. Clin J Pain. 2018;34:878–84.
58. González E, Arias F, Szerman N, et al. Coexistence between personality disorders and substance use disorder. Madrid study about prevalence of dual pathology. Actas Esp Psiquiatr. 2019;47:218–28.

Chapter 3
Prescribing Antidepressant Medication

Where do We Begin?

Most of us have probably been involved in the care of a patient whose story goes something like this:

Miles is a 42-year-old college professor with well-controlled hypertension who comes to see you because he is feeling down. He divorced from his husband a little more than three years ago, and in the last six months he has begun to feel demoralized about what he refers to as "dating in middle age." At the same time, he has been feeling stuck in his career and disappointed with a series of recent failures at work. He can fall asleep at night fairly easily, but often he wakes up around 3:00 am and then lies awake until his alarm goes off at 6:00 am. His energy during the day is low, but he continues to function well enough at work. He has also been losing weight due to both a loss of interest in food and an exercise schedule that strikes you as a bit aggressive. He is still able to enjoy at least a few activities each week, and he denies having any thoughts about suicide.

Your medical assistant administered a PHQ-9 in the waiting room, and his score was a 14, which is consistent with moderate depression. You determine that Miles has major depressive disorder and that a combination of an antidepressant medication and psychotherapy would be appropriate. He agrees to try a medication, although he declines your suggestion of therapy for now, citing a lack of time.

Which Medication Will You Choose?

The answer to this question may be different for everyone. Many factors can go into selecting an antidepressant—desired effects, expected side effects or risks, costs, convenience, drug-drug interactions, other medical comorbidities, or even a well-executed advertising push from a pharmaceutical company [1–4]—but there is inherently some arbitrariness in choosing between agents that are all more or less equally effective. Although some individual research studies have suggested that one medication or another might have a slight edge over its peers in certain circumstances, the preponderance of evidence indicates that, in general, there really are no

© The Author(s), under exclusive license to Springer Nature
Switzerland AG 2022
D. S. Kroll, *Caring for Patients with Depression in Primary Care*,
https://doi.org/10.1007/978-3-031-08495-9_3

significant differences between how likely any one first-line antidepressant medication is to eradicate a patient's depression compared to any others [1, 5, 6].

This does not exactly mean that pulling a medication's name out of hat at random is as good a strategy as any. Although often highly similar in many respects, each medication—and class of medications—has its own individual qualities that may be more or less helpful for any specific patient. If a patient has a personal history of responding favorably to an antidepressant, for example, resuming this previously effective medication is often a good starting point [7]. A family history of a favorable response to a particular medication might similarly point you in this direction.

It is important to note here that taking a family history is not the same as examining underlying genetic factors that may or may not predispose certain patients to good or bad treatment responses. The role of genetic testing in choosing an antidepressant medication is in fact not well established. The genetic testing that is most widely available for this purpose examines specifically whether patients have rapid or slow variants of certain cytochrome P450 isoenzymes—in other words, these tests cannot determine whether or not patients will clinically respond to a certain medication but instead whether higher or lower doses of certain medications will be needed to achieve an optimal effect. 2D6 is the 450 enzyme that is most commonly relevant to the metabolism of antidepressant medications, and its activity is especially likely to impact blood levels of fluoxetine, paroxetine, duloxetine, venlafaxine, and several TCAs. Citalopram and escitalopram levels are more likely to be impacted by 2C19 activity [8].

Individuals who possess an ultrarapid metabolizer (UM) genotype of one or more of these enzymes may be at risk of treatment failure as a result of the medication being cleared too quickly when a usual dosing strategy is used. Thus, a higher dose or more frequent dosing is indicated. Those with a poor metabolizer (PM) genotype, on the other hand, have the opposite problem: the medication is not cleared quickly enough, and a higher risk of medication toxicity ensues [8]. These individuals would benefit from using lower doses or less frequent dosing.

Cytochrome P450 functioning can therefore have significant implications for how some patients respond to typical medication dosing strategies, and some groups have begun to advocate for a more widespread use of genetic testing [9]. However, criticisms of this approach include the fact that how genes affect response to treatment overall remains poorly understood [9]. These tests still cannot tell a patient which medications they should or should not take per se, and their routine use in the selection of antidepressant medications remains controversial, at least at the time of this writing.

Let's start then by going through some key considerations for selecting a medication, both by class and by individual agent:

Selective Serotonin Reuptake Inhibitors (SSRIs)

As a class, SSRIs are used as a default first-line medical treatment for a wide range of depressive and anxiety disorders. They are highly effective and are often considered to be safer and better tolerated than the generation of antidepressants that came

Virtually anything is possible when a human being encounters a new chemical substance for the first time. While this is important to keep in mind when starting any new medication, those that are known to have effects in the central nervous system especially might lead to unpredictable cognitive, emotional, or neurological effects in some individual patients. Acknowledging this unpredictability of response is helpful for both setting patient expectations correctly and addressing underlying fears that an antidepressant medication might "change" someone's personality or make them feel like a "zombie."

Before starting a new antidepressant medication, I often say to patients: "When starting any new medication, it is impossible to predict exactly how it will affect you as an individual. However, the goal of treatment is for you to feel normal—just like you normally would, but without the symptoms of depression. When this is working like it is supposed to, you should feel no difference at all at first (except for any expected good or bad side effects associated with this particular agent), but then gradually—usually at the 4- to 8-week mark—you'll just feel better. It's true that some people describe feeling numb or like a zombie with this medication, but that is not the goal. It is also possible to become more depressed, more agitated, or even suicidal on these medications—these are also not the goal, and they are indications that this medication is not a good fit for you and should be stopped. What we're aiming for with this treatment is just to treat your depression."

Fig. 3.1 Setting treatment expectations and addressing fears about medication

before them, although the idea that their side effects are truly less burdensome than those of the tricyclic antidepressants (TCAs) is not undisputed [5, 10]. They are also especially useful when the depression is comorbid with another psychiatric condition that is similarly responsive to this class of medications, including many anxiety disorders and posttraumatic stress disorder.

SSRIs usually do not exert any therapeutic effects right away (Fig. 3.1). It is common to develop nausea at the beginning of treatment, but this usually resolves fairly quickly [10]. Other common side effects include diarrhea, constipation, headaches (particularly if the patient is already prone to migraines), and sweating [10]. Some patients can also experience dry mouth, tremor, restlessness, increased anxiety, and increased or undesirable dreaming [10]. Sexual side effects are especially common and can include decreased sexual desire, decreased arousal, erectile dysfunction, and a change in orgasm quality (usually for the worse) [2]. Weight gain is possible but not universal, and some individual agents are more problematic than others in this regard [2]. Some (but not all) of the weight gain that occurs with starting an SSRI might also be attributable to reversing the appetite loss that had occurred as a result of the depressive episode [2].

Dosing is usually once per day, and the medication can usually be taken at any time of day depending on patient preference. Some patients experience SSRIs as sedating, and this should prompt them to take their medication at bedtime. Others experience the reverse: they experience their medication as activating and should take it in the morning.

It is also possible for SSRIs to cause new suicidal thoughts to emerge, and this is especially likely in children and in young adults below the age of 24 [1]. If this occurs, the patient should stop taking the new medication immediately, and a suicide risk assessment should be conducted (more on this in Chap. 7). However, suicidal thoughts are not the same as suicidal behaviors or suicide death, and the risk that suicidal thoughts might emerge should not discourage patients from seeking treatment. On the contrary, the overall risk/benefit ratio of using an SSRI to treat depression remains favorable in regard to suicide risk—more often than not, it is better to accept the risk that suicidal thoughts (which can be managed) might occur than to allow the depression to remain untreated [1].

Other medical risks associated with SSRI use, including QTc prolongation, operative bleeding risk, hyponatremia, and serotonin syndrome, will be discussed in Chap. 4.

Here are some characteristics of each SSRI that you might consider when selecting a specific agent, along with their typical therapeutic dosing ranges [1, 2, 8, 10–12]:

Fluoxetine 20–60 mg daily:

- Has the longest half-life of all the SSRIs. It is therefore extremely unlikely to cause withdrawal effects and is more "forgiving" to patients who are prone to skipping doses.
- Is less likely to cause weight gain than other SSRIs.
- Strongly inhibits 2D6 and therefore may interact with other medications that rely on this pathway for their metabolism (e.g., tamoxifen).
- Is most widely available in capsule form, although other forms are also available.

Paroxetine 20–60 mg daily:

- Has the highest affinity among all SSRIs for the serotonin transporter.
- Has stronger anticholinergic effects than other SSRIs and should therefore be avoided in older adults and in patients with glaucoma.
- May cause more severe weight gain and sexual side effects than other SSRIs.
- Should be avoided in pregnancy and breastfeeding.
- Strongly inhibits 2D6.
- Is the most likely of all the SSRIs to cause discontinuation symptoms.

Sertraline 50–200 mg daily:

- Has fewer drug/drug interactions compared to fluoxetine and paroxetine.
- Is associated with a higher incidence of diarrhea compared to other SSRIs.

Citalopram 20–40 mg daily/Escitalopram 10–20 mg daily

- Are more likely to prolong the QTc interval compared to other SSRIs.
- Have a narrower dosing range as a result of an FDA black box warning related to QTc prolongation, and doses higher than 40 mg citalopram/20 mg escitalopram are no longer recommended.
- This dosing range is further capped at 20 mg citalopram/10 mg escitalopram in the presence of other medications that inhibit 2C19 (e.g., omeprazole).
- Citalopram can be given intravenously.
- Escitalopram is exclusively the S-enantiomer of citalopram (literally, S-citalopram), which is thought to be responsible for its therapeutic effects. Any dose of citalopram is therefore therapeutically equivalent to half that dose of escitalopram.

Serotonin Norepinephrine Reuptake Inhibitors (SNRIs)

SNRIs work very similarly to SSRIs except that—as the name implies—they inhibit the reuptake of norepinephrine in addition to serotonin at synapses. Although some early research suggested that they might be slightly more efficacious than SSRIs in the treatment of depression—and thus more useful in severe cases—most studies have found that their efficacies are similar [3]. As a class, their side effects are also similar, although they are more likely to increase blood pressure (particularly venlafaxine) and heart rate [13], and each specific agent has some unique properties.

Prescribers commonly reach for SNRIs as an initial choice for patients who have comorbid chronic pain conditions. These agents have been extensively studied for the purpose of treating chronic pain, and these studies are largely—although not universally—favorable [14–17]. Tricyclic antidepressants (TCAs) appear to be similarly effective [17]. SSRIs and bupropion may also have analgesic effects, but the evidence supporting their use for this purpose is not as robust [17].

Additional considerations with specific agents include the following [3, 13–15, 18–20].

Venlafaxine 75–375 mg daily:

- Comes in both immediate- and extended-release forms. The extended-release form should be used if dosing is given once daily.
- Is more strongly associated with increased diastolic blood pressure compared to other SNRIs.
- Is more likely to cause discontinuation symptoms (Fig. 3.2), sometimes even when once-daily dosing is maintained (in this case, split dosing to twice daily).

SSRIs and SNRIs can cause withdrawal symptoms when they are discontinued too quickly or when doses are skipped (with some agents). Usually, these symptoms are mild and resolve in a matter of days, but in rare cases (particularly with venlafaxine) they can persist for weeks or months. They are not dangerous, but some patients may unintentionally conflate withdrawal symptoms with a recurrence of their depression or anxiety, which has a different clinical presentation. It is important for prescribers to be able to tell the difference between them.

Discontinuation symptoms emerge within a matter of days and can include flu-like symptoms, fatigue, weakness, numbness, tinnitus, dizziness, paresthesias, tremor, myoclonus, pruritis, vision changes, insomnia, cognitive changes, and genital hypersensitivity. Some patients may also describe "electrical" sensations in different parts of the body. Psychiatric symptoms are the most difficult to distinguish from a recurrence of depression but can also include anxiety, depression, and irritability. However, these should still resolve within a few days, and persistent mood or anxiety symptoms beyond this are more likely to signify that the treatment benefit has simply been reversed with removal of the medication.

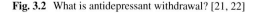

Fig. 3.2 What is antidepressant withdrawal? [21, 22]

Desvenlafaxine 50–100 mg daily:

- Is a metabolite of venlafaxine theorized to have similar therapeutic effects.
- May be associated with lower effectiveness compared to other antidepressant medications.

Duloxetine 30–60 mg twice daily:

- Has been studied for chronic (non-cancer) pain conditions more than other SNRIs and is therefore more commonly used for this purpose.
- Moderately inhibits 2D6.

Levomilnacipran 40–120 mg daily

- Inhibits the reuptake of norepinephrine more strongly than serotonin.
- Is predominantly renally excreted.
- May target low energy and low motivation more directly than other SNRIs and SSRIs.

Bupropion

Bupropion does not have significant serotonergic properties and instead inhibits the reuptake of norepinephrine and dopamine at synapses. It comes in three formulations, which are all equally effective but must be dosed differently. Immediate release bupropion (i.e., "regular" bupropion) is dosed three times daily, sustained release (SR) bupropion is dosed twice daily, and extended-release (XL) bupropion is dosed once daily. The target daily dose for depression is between 300 and 450 mg [3, 23].

Bupropion has stimulant-like effects that can be particularly helpful for patients with low energy or impaired concentration, and it is sometimes used off-label for attention deficit-hyperactivity disorder [24]. It can also lead to weight loss and is FDA-approved for smoking cessation. Possibly because it does not rely on serotonergic properties for its effectiveness, it is also much less likely to cause sexual side effects and is sometimes used in combination with other agents in order to counteract medication-associated sexual dysfunction [25].

Because of its activating effects, bupropion is sometimes avoided in patients who have comorbid anxiety or insomnia, although these are not contraindications, and many individuals with anxiety and insomnia still benefit from it [26]. It can lower the seizure threshold, however, and should be avoided in patients who have seizure disorders or are taking other potentially epileptogenic medications, as well as in patients with anorexia or bulimia [23]. Like some SSRIs, it strongly inhibits 2D6 [3].

Bupropion XL in particular has a reputation for its generic formulation being inferior to the brand-name. This controversy is related to a problem with a single generic formulation of bupropion that was previously used but has since been taken off the market, and at the time of this writing there is no reason to believe that any currently available generic formulations of bupropion are not equivalent to the brand-name [27].

Mirtazapine

Mirtazapine antagonizes a variety of noradrenergic and serotonin receptors and is often referred to as a noradrenergic and specific serotonin antidepressant (NaSSA) [28]. Its therapeutic dosing range is between 15 and 45 mg daily, and it should be taken before bedtime. In addition to its antidepressant effects, its most prominent side effects are sedation and increased appetite [28, 29]. It has a lower risk of causing sexual dysfunction or nausea compared to SSRIs and SNRIs [29].

Although sedation and weight gain may understandably turn off some patients (and prescribers), these side effects can be exploited to help patients who are not sleeping or eating well as part of their depressive symptomatology or as a result of a comorbid medical condition. Mirtazapine also appears to exert antidepressant benefits more quickly than SSRIs and SNRIs, possibly in as few as 2 weeks [29].

Trazodone

Trazodone is a serotonin antagonist and reuptake inhibitor (SARI) that can be dosed at 150–600 mg daily for the treatment of depression. However, it is more commonly used in low doses (12.5–200 mg) off-label as a sedative-hypnotic [30]. It can be heavily sedating and therefore difficult to tolerate when prescribed at its full therapeutic dose for depression, although it is an effective treatment. Other important side effects include orthostatic hypotension, priapism, and QTc prolongation, particularly in overdose [30].

Vilazodone

Vilazodone is a serotonin reuptake inhibitor and partial agonist at the 5HT1A receptor. Its therapeutic dosing range is between 20 and 40 mg daily, and it should be taken with food. Results from early studies claimed that it may be less likely to contribute to sexual dysfunction or weight gain compared to other antidepressants, but this has not been definitively proven [31, 32].

Vortioxetine

Vortioxetine is thought to exert its main effects through a combination of directly modulating serotonin receptor activity while simultaneously inhibiting serotonin transporters, although it affects multiple neurotransmitter systems, and its mechanism of action remains incompletely understood [33, 34]. It is typically dosed between 5 and 20 mg daily. Some studies have suggested that vortioxetine may be less likely to cause sexual dysfunction compared to other antidepressant medications, particularly paroxetine [34]. However, this has not been definitively proven, and its relative strengths and weaknesses compared to other treatments is not yet known [33].

Tricyclic Antidepressants (TCAs)

Though a mainstay of depression treatment for decades, TCAs have largely fallen out of favor as first-line treatments for depression since SSRIs were first introduced [5, 10]. TCAs have a reputation for causing more problematic side effects than more recently developed antidepressants do, and they are far more dangerous in overdose [10]. Nonetheless, they are commonly helpful for other symptoms such as insomnia and many chronic pain conditions, and they remain an effective treatment for depression even if they are considered to be second-line options for most patients.

The therapeutic effects of TCAs are thought to come from reuptake inhibition of serotonin and norepinephrine, whereas their most common side effects mainly stem from their anticholinergic, antihistaminergic, and anti-α-adrenergic properties [10]. Their severity varies from agent to agent, but these side effects include dry mouth, blurry vision, constipation, tachycardia, orthostatic hypotension, and sedation [10]. TCAs are also associated with weight gain (more so than SSRIs), quinidine-like antiarrhythmic effects, and QTc prolongation, particularly in overdose [10]. TCAs should especially be avoided in patients with narrow-angle glaucoma, cognitive impairment, or ventricular rhythm abnormalities or who are taking other class I antiarrhythmic medications or are predictably prone to suicide attempts by overdose [10]. Although commonly also avoided in older patients due to the risk of contributing to confusion and delirium, the fall risk associated with TCAs is similar to that associated with SSRIs [10].

The dosing ranges for TCAs are fairly broad, but many patients benefit from doses that are lower than would traditionally be considered "therapeutic" [35]. While in general, using the lowest effective dose in order to minimize side effects is a good idea, some specific agents are most effective when dosed according to blood levels. Low-dose TCAs are also commonly prescribed (in combination with other antidepressants or not) to directly treat pain or insomnia. Combining two or more serotonergic medications can increase the risk of serotonin toxicity or serotonin syndrome [36], however. This will be discussed in more detail in Chap. 4.

Characteristics that distinguish between some individual TCAs that are still commonly used in practice include the following [36–44]:

Amitriptyline 10–300 mg daily

- Has a stronger serotonergic effect relative to its noradrenergic effect.
- Has potent anticholinergic effects (and therefore side effects).
- Is very commonly used to treat migraine disorders.

Nortriptyline 10–200 mg daily

- Has a stronger noradrenergic effect relative to its serotonergic effect.
- Has weaker anticholinergic effects and milder side effects overall compared to most other TCAs.
- Is less toxic in overdose compared to most other TCAs.
- Has fewer drug-drug interactions compared to most other TCAs.
- Is optimally dosed for depression by following plasma levels. Recommendations for optimum levels vary, but generally they fall in or around the range of 50-150 ng/ml.

Clomipramine 25–250 mg daily

- Has the strongest serotonergic effect among all TCAs and only a weak noradrenergic effect.
- Is commonly used to treat obsessive-compulsive disorder and is used only off-label for depressive disorders.
- May be among the most poorly tolerated of TCAs.
- Can be given intravenously.

Doxepin 10–300 mg daily

- Has very strong antihistaminergic effects (which include sedation and weight gain).
- Is highly sedating and is commonly used in low doses to treat insomnia.
- Is also commonly used to treat pruritus (in both oral and topical forms).

Monoamine Oxidase Inhibitor (MAOIs)

Most patients and prescribers avoid MAOIs due to their unique risk profile and the highly inconvenient dietary restrictions that their use can necessitate. They are generally considered to be appropriate only after other first- and second-line treatments have failed [3, 45]. Nonetheless, they can be highly effective for many patients. They also appear to have a unique benefit for patients who have so-called "atypical" depression features, including increased mood reactivity, prominent anxiety, hypersomnia, increased appetite, and interpersonal rejection sensitivity [3, 46].

As their name implies, MAOIs inhibit monoamine oxidase, an enzyme that is responsible for breaking down serotonin, norepinephrine, dopamine, melatonin and several other neurotransmitters [47]. Tyramine, an amino acid present in certain foods, is one such compound that can accumulate and become highly toxic when an MAOI is used. Tyramine toxicity leads to a hypertensive crisis, which an affected patient might experience as a severe headache, palpitations, and sweating or might rapidly become fatal [3]. For this reason, patients who take MAOIs are advised to

Fig. 3.3 The MAOI diet
[47–49]

> The dietary restrictions recommended for patients who are prescribed MAOIs has been closely scrutinized. Critics argue that the quantity of tyramine in most modern foods is low and that traditional dietary cautions are overly restrictive and inconvenient. Most authors agree that matured, aged, or fermented cheeses and meats, soy sauce and other soy condiments, sauerkraut, fava beans, concentrated yeast extracts, and draft beer should be avoided. All spoiled (or potentially spoiled) foods should also be avoided. Some traditionally excluded foods, including bottled alcohol and pizza (assuming that only fresh cheeses are used) may be safe to consume in moderation.

restrict tyramine-containing foods from their diets (Fig. 3.3). Patients who discover that they have made a dietary indiscretion or who develop symptoms after eating foods that may have contained tyramine are advised to seek treatment in an emergency department [3].

Serotonin syndrome can also occur when an MAOI is combined with another serotonergic medication, including most antidepressants. For this reason, long wash-out periods are required when switching from another antidepressant medication to an MAOI or vice-versa. Most antidepressant medications should be discontinued at least 2 weeks prior to starting an MAOI, and fluoxetine (due to its longer half-life) should discontinued at least 4 weeks beforehand [47]. The antibiotic linezolid also has relatively weak MAOI effects, and it is possible for patients who are taking antidepressant medications to develop serotonin syndrome if they are also treated with this. Combining linezolid with antidepressants is therefore not recommended, although the actual risk appears to be low [50].

MAOIs are also associated with weight gain, sexual dysfunction, dizziness, and myoclonus [3, 51]. Therapeutic doses are typically split into two or three times daily, but starting at the lowest possible dose once daily is usually recommended [3].

Additional considerations related to specific agents include the following [3, 49, 51–55]:

Phenelzine 15–30 mg three times daily

- Has stronger sedating and anti-anxiety effects.
- Is more likely to cause significant weight gain.

Tranylcypromine 10–20 mg three times daily

- Is less sedating and may have an arousing effect.
- Is less likely to contribute to weight gain and sexual side effects.

Isocarboxazid 15–30 mg twice daily

- Has been studied less rigorously than other MAOIs but has also demonstrated efficacy.

Selegiline 6–12 mg daily (transdermal)

- Should be considered for patients who cannot tolerate oral medications.
- Is usually applied to hairless (but not recently shaved) sections of the shoulder, arm, or upper body.
- Application sites should be rotated daily.
- At a dose of 6 mg/day, a low-tyramine diet is not required due to its selective blockade of MAO B.
- At doses of 9 mg/day or higher, a low-tyramine diet is still recommended.

Prescribing Best Practices

One you have selected an agent, the next task is to actually manage the prescription. A common way to do this is simply to prescribe the medication, advise the patient to call with any questions or problems, and ask how things are going at the next follow-up visit, which may occur several weeks or several months later. This is not a very precise method, but the symptoms of depression are inherently difficult to treat algorithmically. As opposed to many other health conditions that are associated with easily observable objective findings, assessing treatment response in depression relies heavily on a patient's self-report at a single point in time, and this can easily be skewed by factors that might contribute to their feeling particularly good or bad on any given day. Traditionally, it is the rule rather than the exception that treatment plans are adjusted or not based on data that can fluctuate widely from day to day and is often unreliable [56]. It is somewhat comparable to trying to manage diabetes mellitus with only sporadic finger stick blood glucose levels to guide you.

The challenge of conducting a follow-up visit for depression can be further illustrated by our case:

Miles returns to see you four weeks after you prescribe sertraline 50 mg daily. He tells you that he is feeling a little better than he did at his last visit, but that had also been at a low point for him, right after a discouraging meeting with his department chair. He is no longer feeling anxious about job security, and a stressful home renovation project has finally ended. He is sleeping a little better, although he continues to feel depressed at times, and he continues to have a bleak outlook on his personal life, but he doesn't see how a medication could fix that.

It is hard to know what to do with this information. Miles's comments suggest that some things have gotten better since the last visit, but a closer look reveals that these pertain to issues that he had not even brought up before, and at the same time, he is implying that he had previously been below his baseline. What you have is essentially an impression of a positive spin on things without a clear demonstration of symptom improvement.

This impression of a positive spin on things can absolutely be consistent with an early therapeutic response to an SSRI. Symptoms improve gradually, and many patients are unable to tell whether or not they are feeling definitively better 4 weeks into treatment. At the same time, this impression can be misleading. Patients may present themselves as doing better than they truly are for a number of reasons, including placebo effects, a desire to please their prescribers, or normal variations in how optimistic they feel from one moment to the next. This has significant implications for the next treatment steps. Patients who are not responding to treatment as they should require adjustments to their treatment plans, and patients who are on track to recovery do not.

There is a real risk that patients who are responding only partially or even minimally to treatment will not have their treatment plans advanced in a timely manner and will therefore remain symptomatic longer than they need to. In other words, they will fall victim to **clinical inertia**. Clinical inertia is a state in which a treatment plan stagnates in the absence of loud or otherwise immediately obvious signals that something is wrong. Patients who continue to have severe, debilitating depression will usually make it clear that their treatment is not working optimally, but those with mild or moderate symptoms often will not. A non-structured approach to follow-up assessments is therefore likely to miss opportunities for treatment plan advancement and lead to slower recovery times and overall poorer outcomes [56].

Clinical inertia is not a problem that is unique to either depression or the primary care setting. However, primary care providers are often treating multiple problems at the same time and cannot reasonably be expected to always probe more deeply after a patient with mild or moderate depression says that they are "better." At the same time, primary care practices are often better prepared to adopt systematic treatment methods than most mental health clinics are because they are more likely to have experience with algorithmic treatment approaches in other areas as well as with population health management and, sometimes, collaborative care.

The solution to overcoming clinical inertia is to use **measurement-based care** [56]. Measurement-based care (or MBC) is the systematic use of a validated symptom rating scale to assess treatment response at regular intervals. In depression, this most commonly means asking patients to complete the nine-item Patient Health Questionnaire (PHQ-9) at the beginning of every visit or, in the case of collaborative care, every two to four weeks.

The PHQ-9 is a nine-item questionnaire that screens for and assesses the severity of the symptoms associated with major depressive disorder. It is useful both as a screening tool and, when used at regular intervals, to assess treatment response. It is not the only scale that is appropriate to use in MBC for depression, but its benefits include that it is brief, easily interpretable, and already widely used in primary care practices.

The benefits to MBC over a non-systematic approach to follow-up assessments are not difficult to imagine. Consider the following two timelines (Figs. 3.4 and 3.5):

The first figure includes only qualitative information that does not lend itself easily to a consistent interpretation over time. Conversely, the second figure provides a clear illustration of how a patient's symptoms have changed since the initiation of treatment and how close they are to their target goals (i.e., clinical remission). MBC takes the guesswork out of applying a patient's often qualitative self-assessment to actionable steps and simultaneously ensures that you do not give up until the target goal has been reached. For these reasons, MBC is strongly associated with better outcomes than usual care and has become the backbone of many high-performing treatment approaches [56].

MBC is not perfect, of course, and using it successfully in the real world is easier said than done. Filling out symptom rating scales can take time, and this time has to come from somewhere. Taking even an extra few minutes out of an already tight clinic schedule can be stressful for clinicians and detract from other agenda items during a visit. Patients would ideally fill out the scales in the (real or virtual) waiting room, but someone has to administer them, and patients who arrive late or cannot complete the scale before the visit start time for any other reason will not benefit

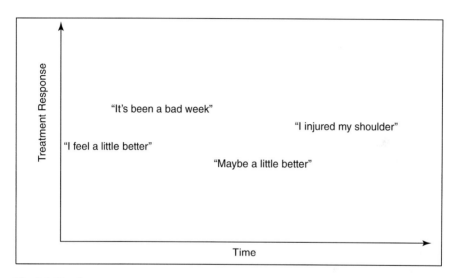

Fig. 3.4 Usual care

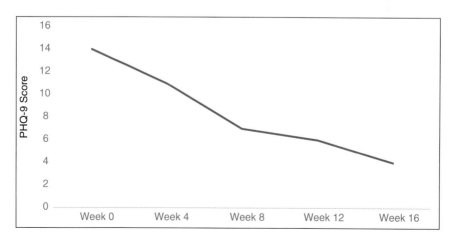

Fig. 3.5 Measurement-based care

from this option. Administering the scale in advance of the visit (e.g., through a patient portal) means giving up some control over how and when the patient completes it, which risks making the information collected by the scales less clinically actionable at the time of the complete assessment.

Several characteristics of a successful MBC approach have been published, however. These include [56]:

– Measurements must be obtained regularly.
– The measurement tools used must be empirically validated (i.e., not homegrown).
– Measurements must be obtained at the time of, or shortly before, clinical encounters to ensure that they are still relevant at the time that care is being provided.
– Clinicians must have the current and any previous measurements readily available at the time of the visit so that they can clinically act (i.e., adjust the treatment plan or not) based on the information contained within them.
– The act of measurement must not create any undue burden on clinicians or clinic staff.

Having an interdisciplinary team who can help to ensure that this information is collected in the correct way can also make a big difference.

After a baseline assessment has been completed, a typical algorithm will prompt prescribing clinicians to start an antidepressant medication at the lowest therapeutic dose and then to use the symptom rating scale to assess whether there has been a reduction in symptoms after four-to-eight weeks of treatment. The dose is then increased if remission has not been achieved (e.g., the PHQ-9 score is still greater than 5), assuming that the patient is not experiencing significant side effects. This process is repeated again after another 4–8 weeks until the patient has taken the maximum therapeutic dose (or the maximum tolerated dose) consistently for 2–3 months. At that point, the patient's score should reflect whether or not the trial has been associated with a meaningful reduction in symptoms and therefore whether it has been successful.

With MBC, most patients can complete a full therapeutic trial of an antidepressant medication within 4–6 months. Its success or failure should inform the next treatment steps:

If a remission has been achieved, no changes are indicated. Patients who have achieved a remission from a first episode of major depressive disorder with an antidepressant medication are typically advised remain on the medication for at least another 4–9 months [3].

If no meaningful reduction in symptoms has been achieved, the medication should be discontinued. This typically involves a gradual taper over several weeks in order to minimize the risk of discontinuation symptoms, or a cross-taper with a different medication. Either way, a different treatment plan should then be initiated, which usually means either a new medication, a referral to psychotherapy, or both.

If some reduction in symptoms has been achieved but not a remission, several options could be considered. A common strategy is to augment the treatment with a second medication that is not an antidepressant or adding a second antidepressant in combination with the first. Augmenting and combining antidepressants will be discussed further in Chap. 6. Alternatively, switching to a different medication entirely could also be considered. A referral to psychotherapy should be strongly considered if it has not been considered already. The overarching rule, however, is that the status quo should not be maintained. Once a therapeutic trial has been completed, new breakthroughs are not expected, and maintaining the treatment plan in its current form is can lead to stagnation.

Switching between Treatments

There are many different ways to switch from one antidepressant medication to another, and there are very few hard and fast rules (except when dealing with MAOIs). However, there is a lower risk of causing discomfort if the medication change is done gradually as opposed to abruptly.

A common way to transition gradually but efficiently from one antidepressant medication to the next is to prescribe a cross-taper. This means gradually decreasing the dose of the first medication at the same time that the second medication is initiated, and then discontinuing the first one as the second one is brought to a therapeutic dose. A typical cross-taper might involve two or three steps that each occur in one-week intervals, but these intervals can be lengthened or shortened depending on the patient's preference and willingness to risk potentially uncomfortable withdrawal symptoms.

For example, consider a patient who has been taking sertraline 100 mg daily for 3 months and is now planning to switch to citalopram 40 mg daily as a result of persistent diarrhea, although sertraline has been effective for her depression. You might suggest the following cross-taper:

- Week 1: sertraline 50 mg daily plus citalopram 20 mg daily.
- Week 2: increase citalopram to 40 mg and stop sertraline.

It would also be reasonable to add a step in between weeks 1 and 2 that involve taking sertraline 25 mg and citalopram 30 mg, particularly if you expect the patient to be more sensitive to the change. Or, if the patient is in a particular rush to stop sertraline as fast as possible, you could make the changes at three-day intervals instead.

In this example, the cross-taper was done between two similar medications at therapeutically equivalent doses, which is relatively easy. However, even if the dosing comparisons are not straightforward, the principle remains the same: gradually reduce one medication while gradually increasing the other.

References

1. Gartlehner G, Hansen RA, Morgan LC, et al. Comparative benefits and harms of second-generation antidepressants for treating major depressive disorder: an updated meta-analysis. Ann Intern Med. 2011;155:772–85.

2. Demyttenaere K, Jaspers L. Bupropion and SSRI-induced side effects. J Psychopharmacol. 2008;22:792–804.
3. American Psychiatric Association. Practice guideline for the treatment of patients with major depressive disorder. 3rd ed; 2010.
4. De las Cuevas C, Sanz EJ, De la Fuente J. Variations in antidepressant prescribing practice: clinical need or market influences? Pharmacoepidemiol Drug Saf. 2002;11:515–22.
5. Undurraga J, Baldessarini RJ. Direct comparison of tricyclic and serotonin-reuptake inhibitor antidepressants in randomized head-to-head trials in acute major depression: systematic review and meta-analysis. J Psychopharmacol. 2017;31:1184–9.
6. Sinyor M, Schaffer A, Levitt A. The sequenced treatment alternatives to relieve depression (STAR*D) Trial: a review. Can J Psychiatr. 2010;55:126–35.
7. Salzman C. Antidepressants. Clin Geriatr Med. 1990;6:399–410.
8. Samer CR, Lorenzini KI, Rollason V, et al. Applications of CYP450 testing in the clinical setting. Mol Diagn Ther. 2013;17:165–84.
9. Bousman CA, Bengesser SA, Aitchison KJ, et al. Review and consensus on pharmacogenomic testing in psychiatry. Pharmacopsychiatry. 2021;54:5–17.
10. Sampson SM. Treating depression with selective serotonin reuptake inhibitors: a practical approach. Mayo Clin Proc. 2001;76:739–44.
11. Uguz F, Sahingoz M, Gungor B, et al. Weight gain and associated factors in patients using newer antidepressant drugs. Gen Hosp Psychiatry. 2015;37:46–8.
12. Nevels RM, Gontkovsky ST, Williams BE. Paroxetine—the antidepressant from hell? Probably not, but caution required. Psychopharmacol Bull. 2016;46:77–104.
13. Carvalho AF, Sharma MS, Brunoni AR, et al. The safety, tolerability and risks associated with the use of newer generation antidepressant drugs: a critical review of the literature. Psychother Psychosom. 2016;85:270–88.
14. Welsch P, Üçeyler N, Klose P, et al. Serotonin and noradrenaline reuptake inhibitors (SNRIs) for fibromyalgia. Cochrane Database Syst Rev. 2018;2:CD010292.
15. Finnerup N, Attal N, Haroutounian S, et al. Pharmacotherapy for neuropathic pain in adults: a systematic review and meta-analysis. Lancet Neurol. 2015;14:162–73.
16. Aiyer R, Barkin RL, Bhatia A. Treatment of neuropathic pain with venlafaxine: a systematic review. Pain Med. 2017;18:1999–2012.
17. Urits I, Peck J, Orhurhu MS, et al. Off-label antidepressant use for treatment and management of chronic pain: evolving understanding and comprehensive review. Curr Pain Headache Rep. 2019;23:66.
18. Loutidis ZG, Kioulos KT. Desvenlafaxine for the acute treatment of depression: a systematic review and meta-analysis. Pharmacopsychiatry. 2015;48:187–99.
19. Katzman MA, Wang X, et al. Effects of desvenlafaxine versus placebo on MDD symptom clusters: a pooled analysis. J Psychopharmacol. 2020;34:280–92.
20. Ragguett R, Yim SJ, Ho PT, McIntyre RS. Efficacy of levomilnacipran extended release in treating major depressive disorder. Expert Opin Pharmacother. 2017;18:2017–24.
21. Davies J, Read J. A systematic review into the incidence, severity and duration of antidepressant withdrawal effects: are guidelines evidence-based? Addict Behav. 2018; https://doi.org/10.1016/j.addbeh.2018.08.027.
22. Fava GA, Gatti A, Belaise C, Guidi J, Offidani E. Withdrawal symptoms after selective serotonin reuptake inhibitor discontinuation: a systematic review. Psychother Psychosom. 2015;84:72–81.
23. Jefferson JW, Pradko JF, Muir KT. Bupropion for major depressive disorder: pharmacokinetic and formulation considerations. Clin Ther. 2005;27:1685–95.
24. Verbeeck W, Bekkeriing GE, Van den Noortgate W, Kramers C. Bupropion for attention deficit hyperactivity disorder (ADHD) in adults. Cochrane Database Syst Rev. 2017;10:CD009504.
25. Zisook S, Rush AJ, Haight BR, et al. Use of bupropion in combination with serotonin reuptake inhibitors. Biol Psychiatry. 2006;59:203–10.

26. Rush AJ, Carmody TJ, Haight BR, et al. Does pretreatment insomnia or anxiety predict acute response to bupropion SR? Ann Clin Psychiatry. 2005;17:1–9.
27. Kharasch ED, Neiner A, Kraus K, et al. Bioequivalence and therapeutic equivalence of generic and brand bupropion in adults with major depressive disorder: a randomized clinical trial. Clin Pharmacol Ther. 2019;105:1164–74.
28. Anttila SAK, Leinonen EVJ. A review of the pharmacological and clinical profile of mirtazapine. CNS Drug Rev. 2001;7:249–64.
29. Watanabe N, Omori IM, Nakagawa A, et al. Mirtazapine versus other antidepressive agents for depression. Cochrane Database Syst Rev. 2011:CD006528.
30. Fagiolini A, Comandini A, Dell'Osso MC, Kasper S. Rediscovering trazodone for the treatment of major depressive disorder. CNS Drugs. 2012;26:1033–49.
31. McCormack P. Vilazodone: a review in major depressive disorder in adults. Drugs. 2015;75:1915–23.
32. Stuivenga M, Giltay EJ, Cools O, et al. Evaluation of vilazodone for the treatment of depressive and anxiety disorders. Expert Opin Pharmacother. 2019;20:251–60.
33. Koesters M, Ostuzzi G, Guaiana G, et al. Vortioxetine for depression in adults. Cochrane Database Syst Rev. 2017;7:CD011520.
34. Jacobsen P, Zhong W, Nomikos G, Clayton A. Paroxetine, but not vortioxetine, impairs sexual functioning compared with placebo in health adults: a randomized, controlled trial. J Sex Med. 2019;10:1638–49.
35. Furukawa TA, McGuire H, Barbui C. Low dosage tricyclic antidepressants for depression. Cochrane Database Syst Rev. 2003;3:CD003197.
36. Gillman PK. Tricyclic antidepressant pharmacology and therapeutic drug interactions updated. Br J Pharmacol. 2007;151:737–48.
37. Burch R. Antidepressants for preventive treatment of migraine. Curr Treat Options Neurol. 2019;21:18.
38. Reynolds CF, Perel JM, Frank E, et al. Three-year outcomes of maintenance nortriptyline treatment in late-life depression: a study of two fixed plasma levels. Am J Psychiatry. 1999;156:1177–81.
39. Ziegler VE, Clayton PJ, Taylor JR, et al. Nortriptyline plasma levels and therapeutic response. Clin Pharmacol Ther. 1976;20:458–63.
40. Cipriani A, Furukawa TA, Salanti G, et al. Comparative efficacy and acceptability of 21 antidepressant drugs for the treatment of adults with major depressive disorder: a systematic review and meta-analysis. Lancet. 2018;391:1357–66.
41. Buoli M, Rovera C, Pzzoli SM, et al. Is trazodone more effective than clomipramine in major depressed outpatients? A single-blind study with intravenous and oral administration. CNS Spectr. 2019;24:258–64.
42. Reddy YCJ, Arumugham SS. Are current pharmacotherapeutic strategies effective in treating OCD? Expert Opin Pharmacother. 2020;21:853–6.
43. Everitt H, Baldwin DS, Stuart B, et al. Antidepressants for insomnia in adults. Cochrane Database Syst Rev. 2018;5:CD010753.
44. Kaur R, Sinha VR. Antidepressants as antipruritic agents: a review. Eur Neuropsychopharmacol. 2018;28:341–52.
45. Suchting R, Tirumalajaru V, Gareeb R, et al. Revisiting monoamine oxidase inhibitors for the treatment of depressive disorders: a systematic review and network meta-analysis. J Affective Disord. 2021;282:1153–60.
46. Parker G, Roy K, Mitchell P, et al. Atypical depression: a reappraisal. Am J Psychiatry. 2002;159:1470–9.
47. Shulman KI, Herrmann N, Walker SE. Current place of monoamine oxidase inhibitors in the treatment of depression. CNS Drugs. 2013;17:789–97.
48. Gillman K. "Much ado about nothing": monoamine oxidase inhibitors, drug interactions, and dietary tyramine. CNS Spectr. 2017;22:385–7.

49. Gillman PK. Advances pertaining to the pharmacology and interactions of irreversible nonse-
    lective monoamine oxidase inhibitors. J Clin Psychopharmacol. 2011;31:66–74.
50. Karkow DC, Kauer FJ, Ernst EJ. Incidence of serotonin syndrome with combined use of
    linezolid and serotonin reuptake inhibitors compared with linezolid monotherapy. J Clin
    Psychopharmacol. 2017;37:518–23.
51. Davidson J, Turnbull C. Isocarboxazid: efficacy and tolerance. J Affect Disord. 1983;5:183–9.
52. Ricken R, Ulrich S, Schlattmann P, Adli M. Tranylcypromine in mind (part II): review
    of clinical pharmacology and meta-analysis of controlled studies in depression. Eur
    Neuropsychopharmacol. 2017;27:714–31.
53. Thase ME, Trivedi MH, Rush AJ. MAOIs in the contemporary treatment of depression.
    Neuropsychopharmacology. 1995;12:185–219.
54. Zisook S. Isocarboxazid in the treatment of depression. Am J Psychiatry. 1983;140:792–4.
55. Cristancho MA, Thase ME. Critical appraisal of selegiline transdermal system for major
    depressive disorder. Expert Opin Drug Deliv. 2016;13:659–65.
56. Fortney JC, Unutzer J, Wrenn G, et al. A tipping point for measurement-based care. Psychiatr
    Serv. 2017;68:179–88.

Chapter 4
Managing Risks and Side Effects of Antidepressant Medications

Even if you have selected a treatment with perfect care, it is still possible to run into problems. Although most antidepressant medications are relatively safe compared to many other classes of drugs used in psychiatry and elsewhere, the risks associated with their use are nonzero, and not every patient responds to them in the way that is intended.

In most cases, it is a good idea to acknowledge this reality at the outset of treatment. While we know that the medications classified as antidepressants have helped millions of people with a variety of psychiatric and other medical conditions, our ability to predict any individual patient's response to a particular treatment remains limited. The range of possible outcomes is wide.

Some undesirable effects are more likely to occur than others, of course. And some involve fairly high stakes. Fortunately, for the most part, they do not overlap too much with the very high-risk ones (with an exception being patients with bipolar disorder—see Fig. 4.1) (Fig. 4.1). In some cases, the side effects we consider to be especially high-risk are also only proximal to—i.e., not the same as—true bad outcomes (e.g., suicidal ideation does not equal a suicide attempt, QTc prolongation does not equal torsades de pointes). Nonetheless, a true bad outcome is truly devastating, and it is important to become familiar with the full range of possibilities that might follow prescribing a medication.

We will therefore start with a discussion of the risks that are most medically serious and how to anticipate and manage them if they emerge. From there, we will move on to the more common side effects that are usually more bothersome than dangerous. This list will not be exhaustive. The possibilities may not be quite infinite, but it would be extraordinarily difficult to include every adverse event that has ever been reported with an antidepressant medication in this chapter and still be able to make sense of this information in the end. Instead, this chapter focuses on the potential adverse effects that are most likely to be relevant to consider and discuss with your patients when selecting a medication, or that patients are likely to ask you about if they emerge (e.g., excessive yawning).

D. S. Kroll, *Caring for Patients with Depression in Primary Care*, https://doi.org/10.1007/978-3-031-08495-9_4

While patients with bipolar disorder are commonly treated with conventional antidepressant medications, this is practice is controversial at best. Antidepressant medications can improve the symptoms of bipolar depression in the short-term, but the potential for benefit is small, and it does not extend to improved remission rates. Meanwhile, there are significant risks, including treatment-emergent mania or hypomania. Even patients who do not experience treatment-emergent manic or hypomanic episodes (and those who are taking other mood stabilizing medications to suppress mania) can experience an acceleration of their depressive cycles—i.e., an increased frequency of depressive episodes—as a result of taking antidepressants.

Because not all patients with bipolar disorder will come to you with this diagnosis already established, there is often a risk that prescribing an antidepressant will unmask a latent bipolar disorder, particularly for patients who are younger and new to treatment. See Chapter 2 for more details about identifying bipolar risk indicators in patients who do not have a history of mania or hypomania.

Fig. 4.1 Special considerations in treating patients with bipolar disorder with antidepressants [1–3]

Suicidal Ideation

Suicidal ideation is perhaps the most dreaded risk that can be associated with virtually all antidepressant medications and one that may cause some prescribers and patients to hesitate before initiating treatment. After the Food and Drug Administration (FDA) first came out with its warning about the risk of suicidal ideation in children and adolescents in 2003 and extended it to young adults in 2007, antidepressant prescription rates in fact declined for both children and adults in many countries [4–6]. An associated finding was that over the same time frame, suicide death rates increased [4, 6]. While it was never scientifically proven that the FDA's decision created a new barrier to treatment or otherwise directly or indirectly contributed to the increased frequency of suicide deaths over this period, this observation has nonetheless opened the door to criticism about the warning. At the very least, it highlights the concern that the FDA's warning about the risk of suicidality associated with antidepressant medication should not be simply accepted as a headline but rather understood in context.

The FDA's actual language on this issue is not terribly provocative and likely was not intended to discourage treatment. It states:

Antidepressants increased the risk compared to placebo of suicidal thinking and behavior (suicidality) in children, adolescents, and young adults in short-term studies of major depressive disorder (MDD) and other psychiatric disorders. Anyone considering the use of [Insert established name] or any other antidepressant in a child, adolescent, or young adult must balance this risk with the clinical need. Short-term studies did not show an increase in the risk of suicidality with antidepressants compared to placebo in adults beyond age 24; there was a reduction in risk with antidepressants compared to placebo in adults aged 65 and older. Depression and certain other psychiatric disorders are themselves associated with increases in the risk of suicide. Patients of all ages who are started on antidepressant therapy should be monitored appropriately and observed closely for clinical worsening, suicidality, or unusual changes in behavior [7].

None of this is disputable. Suicidal ideation can emerge following the initiation of an antidepressant medication in any patient, and this appears to be significantly more common in patients who are under the age of 25. The cause of this finding is not well understood, but potential explanations as to why suicidality should occur more often in younger patients taking antidepressants include a higher likelihood of their having a latent bipolar disorder (remember that bipolar disorder typically presents at a younger age, and depressive episodes may precede manic or hypomanic episodes), the likelihood that human brains may respond differently to certain somatic treatments at different stages of development, age-related differences in metabolism, and higher risks of impulsivity and substance use at younger ages [4].

Whatever the true cause of this association may be, another important fact should not get lost: *the most effective way to mitigate suicide risk is to treat the underlying depression* [4, 8, 9]! In other words, even though suicidal thoughts might emerge in the context of treatment, neglecting to treat depression is associated with a greater overall risk of a patient's dying by suicide.

Although it is more common among children and adolescents, medication-associated suicidal ideation can occur at any age. Typically, it emerges within the first few days or weeks of beginning treatment, or shortly after a dose increase [8]. The vast majority of cases involving antidepressant-associated suicidal ideation do not progress to suicide attempts, and suicide death in this context is extremely rare [4, 8, 10]. Nonetheless, this risk requires some attention.

First, it is important to assess suicide risk at the outset of treatment. A suicide risk assessment is a necessary part of any psychiatric diagnostic assessment regardless of the treatment under consideration, and specific strategies for doing this will be described in detail in Chap. 7. However, in this context is it particularly relevant for establishing a baseline and anticipating whether additional supports should be mobilized. A safety plan should also be discussed and documented (more on this in Chap. 7).

After the medication has been prescribed, it is a good idea to check in with the patient approximately 1 week later, and then again at one-week intervals for the next few weeks if possible [4]. This does not require face-to-face visits; calling the patient, or asking a nurse or social worker on your team to call the patient, is usually adequate. Since treating depression is a team sport, so to speak, having a standard protocol that deliberately involves other team members at this stage can be especially helpful in reinforcing the importance of team-based care to the patient. Whoever calls the patient should inquire about suicidal ideation and also screen for any other treatment-emergent side effects that could be associated with suicidal behavior, including agitation, insomnia, or mania [4]. While agitation and insomnia can be addressed with further treatment, the presence of new or significantly worsening suicidal ideation or mania should prompt you to discontinue the medication immediately, reassess the risk level, and reinforce the safety plan [4]. The presence of suicidal ideation alone does not necessarily warrant hospitalization, but this can be considered in cases of especially high risk or inadequate support.

Serotonin Syndrome

Medical providers are often taught about serotonin syndrome based on the way it presents in emergency departments: altered mental status, neuromuscular rigidity, hyperthermia, and autonomic changes leading to a high risk of mortality. While this is not inaccurate—serotonin syndrome can certainly be fatal—thinking about serotonin syndrome as something that exists only in its fulminant form can lead ambulatory providers to miss cases.

It is helpful to think about serotonin syndrome as another label for serotonin toxicity [11]. Any mechanisms (which are usually iatrogenic) that increase serotonergic activity within the central and peripheral nervous systems can overshoot the mark and produce toxic symptoms. In mild cases, this may even be difficult to differentiate from more routine medication side effects or untreated psychiatric symptoms—for example, tremor, anxiety, restlessness, insomnia, gastrointestinal upset, and diaphoresis [12, 13]. However, in cases of true serotonin toxicity, these symptoms are likely to progress (unless the offending treatment is discontinued) and are likely to include other telltale findings on examination, including tachycardia, hypertension, hyperthermia, hyperreflexia, mydriasis, myoclonus, clonus, and hyperactive bowel sounds [12]. In severe cases, extreme muscle rigidity leads to severe hyperthermia, which in turn can lead to organ failure, along with hemodynamic instability, seizures, delirium, coma, and death [13]. Of course, this is how it becomes a medical emergency.

It is possible for a patient to develop serotonin syndrome even from taking a single antidepressant medication at a therapeutic dose [13]. At the same time, it is possible to take multiple antidepressant medications together at high doses and never develop signs of toxicity. There is no specific threshold of serotonergic medication that is known to differentiate high- from low-risk combinations (with the exception of combinations involving MAOIs, which are much more commonly forbidden). Instead, we are left with guidelines and warnings.

As a general rule, however, *medications and combinations that result in a stronger serotonergic effect are more likely to result in serotonin toxicity*. While this seems obvious on paper, it may not be in practice. Medical (and some nonmedical) substances can increase serotonergic activity in a number of different ways [12]. Most of the commonly used antidepressant medications reduce presynaptic serotonin reuptake or act as agonists at postsynaptic serotonin receptors. MAOIs prevent serotonin breakdown, often irreversibly, which is why it is especially dangerous to combine them with other serotonergic agents. Central nervous system stimulants and other amphetamines directly increase serotonin release. Some agents (such as tryptophan) can lead to increased production of serotonin, whereas any substance that inhibits P450 enzymes (particularly 2D6 or 3A4) could delay its metabolism.

For these reasons, it is a good idea not to go overboard with prescribing serotonergic medications. Stay within therapeutic dosing ranges (unless you have identified a specific reason to exceed these ranges—e.g., an ultrarapid metabolizer phenotype for P450 enzymes), and avoid combining multiple agents that have serotonergic effects if possible. This does not mean that it is never safe to combine two or more serotonergic medications—SSRI/TCA combinations are extremely common in patients with pain conditions, for example, and the vast majority of patients who take triptan drugs for migraines along with antidepressants do not develop serotonin toxicity [11, 14]. However, if combining medications is necessary, keep in mind that low doses pose lower risks than high doses do, and two-drug combinations are safer than multi-drug combinations. As polypharmacy increases in general, the risk that more insidious mechanisms (e.g., P450 inhibition) could be overlooked also becomes higher. For example, the risk associated with combining a therapeutic dose of an SSRI with 10-25 mg nightly of amitriptyline or 25–50 mg nightly of trazodone is significantly different from the risk associated with combining a therapeutic dose of an SSRI with 120 mg daily of duloxetine and 200 mg nightly of trazodone along with ondansetron and tramadol. But the risk associated with either of these combinations is still greater than zero.

Bleeding

Medications that inhibit serotonin reuptake (e.g., SSRIs, SNRIs) impair platelet functioning by depleting platelets of serotonin [15]. At the same time, untreated depression is associated with increased platelet activity and a hypercoagulable state, which may underlie the increased risk of coronary artery disease and stroke that patients with depression face [15].

There is therefore some balance between the good and bad effects of SSRIs' and SNRIs' antiplatelet activity, which is thought to be comparable to that of aspirin [15]. This may even be one of the mechanisms by which antidepressant treatment reduces myocardial infarction risk and mortality among patients with ischemic heart disease [15]. Nonetheless, patients who take SSRIs and SNRIs have an increased risk of bleeding events, particularly in the upper gastrointestinal system [15].

Consensus guidelines around when to avoid or discontinue an antidepressant medication in situations that involve a higher risk of bleeding (such as surgery) are lacking. Instead, prescribers are advised to use their own clinical judgment regarding the relative risks and benefits for their patients [15].

QTc Prolongation

Some antidepressant medications—particularly TCAs, trazodone, citalopram, and escitalopram—can prolong the QTc interval in a dose-dependent manner [16–18]. Other SSRIs, SNRIs, and mirtazapine have also been associated with QTc prolongation to a lesser degree, but the clinical significance of these associations, if any, is not well established [16, 17, 19]. Bupropion has been associated with QTc prolongation in overdose but may actually shorten the QTc interval at therapeutic doses [20, 21].

No specific recommendations regarding the use of ECG monitoring in patients who are taking antidepressant medications at therapeutic doses have been developed. Evidence-based guidelines around which patients should or should not avoid taking antidepressant medications out of concern for the risk of developing a fatal cardiac arrhythmia are similarly lacking, but the FDA specifically warns against the use of citalopram for patients who are already at risk of ventricular arrhythmias or who already have a prolonged QTc interval [22]. The FDA also advises against prescribing citalopram at doses higher than 20 mg per day for patients who are over the age of 60 or are taking other medications that can inhibit 2C19 (such as cimetidine and omeprazole) [22].

Hyponatremia

Hyponatremia is a potentially serious side effect of most antidepressant medications with an incidence that is not well-established, in part because it has not been studied extensively and in part because not all of the studies that exist define hyponatremia in the same way [23, 24]. Studies that have defined hyponatremia by a serum concentration of less than 135 mmol/L have, not surprisingly, found that it has a higher incidence than those that defined it by a concentration of less than 130 mmol/L [24].

It appears to be more strongly associated with SSRIs than with other antidepressant classes [23, 24]. It also more commonly occurs in women, patients who have other medical comorbidities, and older patients, particularly if they are taking other medications that can reduce sodium levels [24]. Older patients in particular are more likely to develop cognitive impairment, falls, and osteoporosis as a result of their sodium levels being low [23].

Hepatotoxicity

Severe hepatotoxicity related to antidepressant medication use is extremely rare, except in the case of nefazodone, a medication that has been removed from the United States market as a result of this risk [25, 26]. Antidepressant-associated liver toxicity typically presents as an asymptomatic elevation in serum transaminases; but severe, irreversible injury and fulminant hepatic failure are possible [26]. Onset appears to be highest within the first 6 months of treatment [26].

Agents that are more strongly associated with liver injury include duloxetine, bupropion, trazodone, and amitriptyline [26]. Conversely, citalopram, escitalopram, and paroxetine appear to be safer in this regard [26]. Formal guidelines around how to anticipate and mitigate this risk are lacking, but some authors recommended checking liver function tests at baseline and at regular intervals, particularly for older adults or for patients who have other risk factors for hepatic injury, such as alcohol use disorders and polypharmacy [25, 26].

Falls and Fractures

Both depression and the use of antidepressant medications has been associated with a higher risk of falls, particularly in older adults [10, 27]. Multiple mechanisms may contribute to this, including orthostatic hypotension and bradycardia that are directly related to class of medication as well as other medications that patients with depression commonly take (e.g., benzodiazepines) [10]. At the same time, both SSRIs and major depressive disorder have been associated with decreased bone density and a higher risk of fractures.

How this association should impact treatment decisions remains unknown [25, 28]. It is not clear that different classes of antidepressants are more or less safe in regard into either fall risk or osteoporosis, and avoiding antidepressant treatment entirely in patients who are depressed and may have an especially high risk of fractures is not recommended [28]. Instead, the specific risks of each individual case should be considered, and other steps to mitigate the risks of fractures and falls, such as lifestyle improvements and reducing polypharmacy, should also be taken [28].

Seizures

Bupropion can lower the seizure threshold and is generally not recommended for patients with epilepsy or who are otherwise at an elevated risk of seizures [29]. It is also especially likely to induce seizures in patients with bulimia nervosa, and it is generally considered to be contraindicated in both bulimia nervosa and anorexia nervosa (in part because it also suppresses the appetite and can exacerbate weight loss) [10, 29]. Some patients can develop seizures while taking bupropion even if they do not have any underlying risks and are taking it at a therapeutic dose [29]. Guidelines therefore recommend that doses never exceed 450 mg per day, are uptitrated gradually, and are divided for IR and SR formulations (but not the XR) [10].

SSRIs and SNRIs can also cause seizures in cases of overdose or toxicity, but they are not clearly associated with a heightened seizure risk at therapeutic doses [30]. There is a stronger association between seizure risk and the TCAs clomipramine and amoxapine as well as the tetracyclic antidepressant maprotiline [30].

None of these risks should deter treatment for most patients. Instead, awareness of them may guide you to preferentially select some medication classes over others for patients who have specific health conditions or risks, and to monitor for potentially emerging risk indicators where applicable. Most patients who take antidepressant medications will not be clinically affected by these and are far more likely to experience one or more of the following, which are not likely to result in medical emergencies.

Sexual Dysfunction

While impaired sexual functioning is often multifactorial and can even be a result of depression itself, the link between several classes of antidepressants—including SSRIs, SNRIs, TCAs, and MAOIs—and sexual side effects is indisputable [31]. Impaired sexual functioning may occur in as many as 80% of patients who are treated with SSRIs and typically involve negative effects on sexual desire, arousal, and/or orgasm but can also include impotence [32, 33]. The importance of this varies from patient to patient, but in some cases, sexual dysfunction can become so problematic (e.g., by damaging a patient's self-esteem or causing relationship conflicts) that it interferes with recovery from depression [31].

It is possible that sexual side effects from an antidepressant medication will resolve spontaneously after several months [33]. However, watchful waiting does not work in most cases, and not all patients are willing to wait. Fortunately, many other strategies for mitigating sexual side effects can be considered. These include:

Try a lower dose. Lowering doses often results in a lower severity of severe side effects. The limiting factor in this strategy is, of course, that a lower dose may also be less effective as a treatment for depression.

Try a different medication. Bupropion and mirtazapine are much less likely to cause sexual side effects than other commonly prescribed antidepressants, and if all other factors (including efficacy) are equal, a switch may work very well. Even within classes, some agents are more likely to cause sexual side effects than others, typically correlating with the strength of its serotonergic properties (e.g., among SSRIs, paroxetine is especially likely to cause sexual side effects) [33]. A trial of a newer medication, such as vortioxetine or vilazodone, can also be considered, although it is too early to say whether the claims that these agents are less likely to cause sexual dysfunction will stand the test of time (at least at the time of this writing) [34, 35].

Augment treatment with another medication that may offset sexual side effects. Adjunctive bupropion can reduce the sexual dysfunction associated with other antidepressant medications in both men and women [31, 33]. Pimavanserin, an antipsychotic medication that is also an inverse agonist at serotonin receptors, may similarly improve sexual functioning [36]. Phosphodiesterase type 5 such as sildenafil have a stronger track record for improving arousal in men but may still be helpful for increasing the intensity of orgasm in women [31, 33].

Change the timing or frequency of dosing. Drug holidays, particularly for agents with a short half-life, can be considered around a patient's plans for engaging in sexual activity. There are risks to this approach, including precipitating withdrawal symptoms and disrupting treatment, and therefore it is not usually considered to be a first-line option [31, 33]. Dosing the medication after sex may also help in some cases, particularly if the medication has a short half-life [31].

Try behavioral management. Several behavior adaptations have also shown to be helpful, particularly in women. These include scheduling sex, exercising immediately before sex, and using a vibrator for stimulation [33].

Although sexual side effects usually also resolve completely when the offending medication is discontinued, some patients continue to report persistent sexual dysfunction afterward [37]. The frequency of this phenomenon is unknown, and it remains poorly understood [37].

Gastrointestinal Side Effects

Nausea and vomiting are among the most common side effects that emerge at the beginning of treatment with antidepressant medications, particularly SSRIs and SNRIs [25, 38]. These symptoms usually resolve spontaneously with continued treatment but may persist in some cases [38]. Diarrhea can similarly persist and is most closely associated with sertraline [9].

Mirtazapine is unique in this regard as it is relatively unlikely to cause nausea or vomiting and may even be useful as an antiemetic in some cases [39, 40].

Weight Changes

Weight gain in the context of treating depression is usually multifactorial, and obesity correlates with depression regardless of treatment [41]. Some of the weight gain that occurs with antidepressant medication may also be attributable to reversing the appetite loss associated with treatment [32]. However, this is a recognized risk of many antidepressant medications.

Mirtazapine is the agent that is most likely to cause weight gain because it directly stimulates the appetite [25]. Conversely, bupropion typically suppresses the appetite and can cause weight loss [25, 42]. The risk of weight gain may be higher in younger patients and in those who have sedentary lifestyles [41].

Effects on Sleep

Trazodone, mirtazapine, and most TCAs (except desipramine) can cause sedation and may improve sleep in many patients [25, 43]. These should usually be dosed at bedtime in order to maximize the benefit from this effect.

SSRIs and SNRIs can cause either insomnia or somnolence depending on the individual patient, and this may inform whether the patient doses these medications in the morning or at night [43]. Bupropion has a stimulating effect on the central nervous system and is more likely to cause insomnia [43].

SSRIs and SNRIs can occasionally disrupt sleep in other ways by causing vivid dreams or nightmares [25]. SSRIs, SNRIs, and mirtazapine can also exacerbate restless legs syndrome [25].

Activation and Anxiety

Initial treatment with SSRIs and some other antidepressants is sometimes associated with increased anxiety, physical activity, and/or restlessness [10, 44, 45]. The symptoms that can be attributed to this "activation syndrome" are highly heterogeneous and include anxiety, panic attacks, insomnia, irritability, aggressiveness, impulsivity, mania, and suicidal ideation [44]. It is therefore likely that the designation of an activation syndrome may represent a number of different processes that could follow the initiation of an antidepressant medication.

The emergence of new suicidal ideation or mania warrants immediate discontinuation of treatment, but milder anxiety or arousal symptoms may resolve or improve over time [10, 44]. Temporary use of beta-blocker or benzodiazepine may help in some cases [10]. Starting the antidepressant medication at low doses may also mitigate this risk [10].

Emotional Detachment

Some patients who take antidepressant medications report a persistent feeling of emotional blunting or detachment that is separate from their depressive symptoms [32]. They may complain of numbness, apathy, fatigue, or feeling "like a zombie." It is important to reassure such patients that emotional numbness is not the goal of treatment, and the presence of this treatment side effect should not be construed to mean that no medication will ever work for them. Switching to a different treatment plan (either another antidepressant medication or a different modality of treatment) should be discussed, although some patients may prefer to continue their current treatment depending on the severity of their depression and whether or not the medication has otherwise been effective.

Headaches

It seems like a paradox that headaches are listed as a potential side effect of virtually all antidepressant medications, and yet many antidepressant medications are used specifically to treat headache disorders [46]. And yet, it is common for patients to report either new-onset headaches or an exacerbation of a pre-existing headache condition shortly after starting treatment.

The extent to which antidepressant medications truly induce headaches seems to vary by class. Bupropion and trazodone carry a higher risk of causing headaches than SSRIs, which in turn carry only a slightly higher risk of causing headaches compared to placebo [46]. SNRIs and TCAs are unlikely to cause or exacerbate headaches [46]. Headaches that are related to antidepressant treatment typically resolve spontaneously after a few weeks of starting treatment, and long-term use of many antidepressants—including SSRIs, SNRIs, TCAs, and mirtazapine—is associated with an overall favorable impact on the course of headache disorders [10, 46, 47].

Diaphoresis

Excessive sweating is associated with SSRIs, SNRIs, TCAs, and bupropion [25]. There is limited evidence that adjunctive benztropine or cyproheptadine may mitigate this side effect [25].

Yawning

SSRIs and SNRIs have been associated with excessive yawning, independently from excessive sleepiness [48]. The clinical importance of this is likely to vary between patients, but some may choose to discontinue or switch their medications as a result.

It is worth reiterating that antidepressant medications, for the most part, are safe to use in the vast majority of patients. Like any other type of medical treatment, they do not work perfectly in everyone and can do more harm than good some of the time. However, this fact should not universally deter treatment. The benefits of treating depression usually outweigh the risks.

Medications are not the only solution, however. In the next chapter, we will discuss the other mainstay of treating depression, psychotherapy. Choosing psychotherapy over medication allows patients to dispense with iatrogenic medical complications altogether, but as you will soon see, this treatment is not entirely without risks or complications, either.

References

1. Ghaemi SN. Why antidepressants are not antidepressants: STEP-BD, STAR*D, and the return of neurotic depression. Bipolar Disord. 2008;10:957–68.
2. McGirr A, Vöhringer PA, Ghaemi SN, et al. Safety and efficacy of adjunctive second-generation antidepressant therapy with a mood stabilizer or an atypical antipsychotic in acute

bipolar depression: a systematic review and meta-analysis of randomized placebo-controlled trials. Lancet. Psychiatry. 2016;3:1138–46.

3. Benvenuti A, Rucci P, Miniati M, et al. Treatment-emergent mania/hypomania in unipolar patients. Bipolar Disord. 2008;10:726–32.
4. Brent DA. Antidepressants and suicidality. Psychiatr Clin North Am. 2016;39:503–12.
5. Katz LY, Kozyrskyj AL, Prior JH, et al. Effect of regulatory warnings on antidepressant pre-scription rates, use of health services and outcomes among children, adolescents and young adults. CMAJ. 2008;178:1005–11.
6. Libby AM, Orton HD, Valuck RJ. Persisting decline in depression treatment after FDA warn-ings. Arch Gen Psychiatry. 2009;66:633–9.
7. Food and Drug Administration. Revisions to product labeling. https://www.fda.gov/media/77404/download. Accessed 5/12/21 10:04am.
8. Stübner S, Grohmann R, Greil W, et al. Suicidal ideation and suicidal behavior as rare adverse events of antidepressant medication: current report from the AMSP multicenter drug safety surveillance project. Int J Neuropsychopharmacol. 2018;21:814–21.
9. Gartlehner G, Hansen RA, Morgan LC, et al. Comparative benefits and harms of second-generation antidepressants for treating major depressive disorder: an updated meta-analysis. Ann Intern Med. 2011;155:772–85.
10. American Psychiatric Association. Practice guideline for the treatment of patients with major depressive disorder. 3rd ed; 2010.
11. Gillman PK. Tricyclic antidepressant pharmacology and therapeutic drug interactions updated. Br J Pharmacol. 2007;151:737–48.
12. Wang RZ, Vashistha V, Kaur S, Houchens NW. Serotonin syndrome: preventing, recognizing, and treating it. Cleve Clin J Med. 2016;83:810–7.
13. Boyer EW, Shannon M. The serotonin syndrome. N Engl J Med. 2005;352:1112–20.
14. Orlova Y, Rizzoli P, Loder E. Association of coprescription of triptan antimigraine drugs and selective serotonin reuptake inhibitor or selective norepinephrine reuptake inhibitor antide-pressants with serotonin syndrome. JAMA Neurol. 2018;75:566–72.
15. Roose SP, Rutherford BR. Selective serotonin reuptake inhibitors and operative bleeding risk: a review of the literature. J Clin Psychopharmacol. 2016;36:704–9.
16. Beach SR, Kostis WJ, Celano CM, et al. Meta-analysis of selective serotonin reuptake inhibitor-associated QTc prolongation. J Clin Psychiatry. 2014;75:e441-9.
17. Hasnain M, Vieweg WVR. QTc interval prolongation and torsade de pointes associated with second-generation antipsychotics and antidepressants: a comprehensive review. CNS Drugs. 2014;28:887–920.
18. Tellone V, Rosignoli MT, Picollo R, et al. Effect of 3 single doses of trazodone on QTc interval in health subjects. J Clin Pharmacol. 2020;60:1483–95.
19. Gurkan S, Liu F, Chain A, Gutstein DE. A study to assess the proarrhythmic potential of mirtazapine using concentration-QTc (C-QTc) analysis. Clin Pharmacol Drug Dev. 2019;8:449–58.
20. Jasiak NM, Bostwick JR. Risk of QT/QTc prolongation among newer non-SSRI antidepres-sants. Ann Pharmacother. 2013;48:1620–8.
21. Castro VM, Clements CC, Murphy SN, et al. QTc interval and antidepressant use: a cross-sectional study of electronic health records. BMJ. 2013;346:f288.
22. Food and Drug Administration. FDA Drug Safety Communication: revised recommendations for Celexa (citalopram hydrobromide) related to a potential risk of abnormal heart rhythms with high doses. https://www.fda.gov/drugs/drug-safety-and-availability/fda-drug-safety-communication-revised-recommendations-celexa-citalopram-hydrobromide-related. Revised 12/15/17. Accessed 5/16/21 at 12:21pm.
23. Leth-Møller KB, Hansen AH, Torstensson M, et al. Antidepressants and the risk of hyponatre-mia: a Danish register-based population study. BMJ Open. 2016;6:e011200.
24. De Picker L, Van Den Eede F, Dumont G, et al. Antidepressants and the risk of hyponatremia: a class-by-class review of literature. Psychosomatics. 2014;55:536–47.

25. Carvalho AF, Sharma MS, Brunoni AR, et al. The safety, tolerability and risks associated with the use of newer generation antidepressant drugs: a critical review of the literature. Psychother Psychosom. 2016;85:270–88.
26. Voican CS, Corruble E, Naveau S, Perlemuter G. Antidepressant induced liver injury: a review for clinicians. Am J Psychiatry. 2014;171:404–15.
27. Lohman MC, Fairchild AJ, Merchant AT. Antidepressant use partially mediates the association between depression and risk of falls and fall injuries among older adults. J Gerontol A Biol Sci Med Sci. 2020:glaa253.
28. Power C, Duffy R, Mahon J, et al. Bones of contention: a comprehensive literature review of non-SSRI antidepressant use and bone health. J Geriatr Psychiatry Neurol. 2020;33:340–52.
29. Dwoskin LP, Rauhut AS, King-Pospisil KA, Bardo MT. Review of the pharmacology and clinical profile of bupropion, an antidepressant and tobacco use cessation agent. CNS Drug Rev. 2006;12:178–207.
30. Kanner AM. Most antidepressant drugs are safe for patients with epilepsy at therapeutic doses: a review of the evidence. Epilepsy Behav. 2016;61:282–6.
31. Segraves RT, Balon R. Antidepressant-induced sexual dysfunction in men. Pharmacol Biochem Behav. 2014;121:132–7.
32. Demyttenaere K, Jaspers L. Bupropion and SSRI-induced side effects. J Psychopharmacol. 2008;22:792–804.
33. Lorenz T, Rullo J, Faubion S. Antidepressant-induced female sexual dysfunction. Mayo Clin Proc. 2016;91:1280–6.
34. Koesters M, Ostuzzi G, Guaiana G, et al. Vortioxetine for depression in adults. Cochrane Database Syst Rev. 2017;7:CD011520.
35. Stuivenga M, Giltay EJ, Cools O, et al. Evaluation of vilazodone for the treatment of depressive and anxiety disorders. Expert Opin Pharmacother. 2019;20:251–60.
36. Freeman MP, Fava M, Dirks B, et al. Improvement of sexual functioning during treatment of MDD with adjunctive pimavanserin: a secondary analysis. Depress Anxiety. 2020;37:485–95.
37. Bala A, Nguyen HMT, Hellstrom WJG. Post-SSRI sexual dysfunction: a literature review. Sex Med Rev. 2018;6:29–34.
38. Sampson SM. Treating depression with selective serotonin reuptake inhibitors: a practical approach. Mayo Clin Proc. 2001;76:739–44.
39. Watanabe N, Omori IM, Nakagawa A, et al. Mirtazapine versus other antidepressive agents for depression. Cochrane Database Syst Rev. 2011:CD006528.
40. Cangemi DJ, Kuo B. Practical perspectives in the treatment of nausea and vomiting. J Clin Gastroenterol. 2019;53:170–8.
41. Gafoor R, Booth HP, Gulliford MC. Antidepressant utilization and incidence of weight gain during 10 years' follow-up: population based cohort study. BMJ. 2018;351:k1951.
42. Alonso-Pedrero L, Bes-Rastrollo M, Marti A. Effects of antidepressant and antipsychotic use on weight gain: a systematic review. Obes Rev. 2019;20:1680–90.
43. Mayers AG, Baldwin DS. Antidepressants and their effect on sleep. Hum Psychopharmacol. 2005;20:533–59.
44. Harada Y, Sakamoto K, Ishigooka J. Incidence and predictors of activation syndrome induced by antidepressants. Depress Anxiety. 2008;25:1014–9.
45. Bussing R, Reid AM, McNamara JPH, et al. A pilot study of actigraphy as an objective measure of SSRI activation symptoms: results from a randomized placebo controlled psychopharmacological treatment study. Psychiatry Res. 2015;225:440–5.
46. Telang S, Walton C, Olten B, Bloch MH. Meta-analysis: second generation antidepressants and headache. J Affect Disord. 2018;236:60–8.
47. Jackson JL, Mancuso JM, Nickoloff S, et al. Tricyclic and tetracyclic antidepressants for the prevention of frequent episodic or chronic tension type headache in adults: a systematic review and meta-analysis. J Gen Intern Med. 2017;32:1351–8.
48. Hensch T, Blume A, Böttger D, et al. Yawning in depression: worth looking into. Pharmacopsychiatry. 2015;48:118–20.

Chapter 5
Referring to Therapy

It almost always helps to talk to someone—or, at least, we think so. The idea that psychotherapy is helpful for patients with depression can almost be taken for granted—in some respects, it is not all that different from saying that physical therapy is an integral part of recovery after surgery or that patients with diabetes would benefit from working with a dietician. Most patients with virtually any psychiatric condition will get better outcomes if therapy is a part of their treatment.

And yet, referring to psychotherapy doesn't always work. Why? Consider the following case, which may be all too familiar:

Gail is a 38-year-old mother of two children who first reported to you that she was feeling depressed 6 months ago, shortly after her youngest daughter was diagnosed with a developmental disorder. She was married, but her husband drove a tractor-trailer for a living and was rarely home. Meanwhile, she was working from home part-time as a customer service representative while her children were in school, but this job was not very rewarding, nor was it particularly flexible or accommodating when her children were at home, which often caused "trouble," to use her words. She was feeling depressed most of the time and had difficulty thinking of anything in her life that she enjoyed, although her family had recently thrown her a surprise party for her birthday, and she had felt genuinely moved by this. She was sleeping about 6 hours per night and feeling lethargic most of the day. She was overeating—mostly junk food because she didn't have time to cook—and had gained about fifteen pounds in the prior year.

When you first addressed her condition 6 months ago, you diagnosed an adjustment disorder and discussed a plan to start with psychotherapy before considering medication. She seemed eager to try this, and you asked a resource specialist in your practice to provide her with a list of therapists in her area who accepted her insurance...

Perhaps you can see where this story is going. Of course, one would hope that when Gail returns for her follow-up visit with you, she will say that she successfully connected with one of the therapists on her list and that she has already begun to feel

D. S. Kroll, *Caring for Patients with Depression in Primary Care*, https://doi.org/10.1007/978-3-031-08495-9_5

more confident and focused on the problems in her life, and meanwhile she has ditched her predatory customer service job and found a better one within her daughter's school that allows her to be more accessible during the day and also makes it easier for her to know about and advocate for the right resources. But so many things could have gone wrong along the way. Maybe she never received the list from your resource specialist. Maybe she never tried calling any of the therapists on the lists, or maybe she did, but none of the therapists returned her call. Maybe some of the therapists did return her call, but they could not or would not give Gail a straight answer about whether her insurance would actually pay for the treatment, and Gail became demoralized. Maybe she did meet with a therapist, but she didn't feel much of a connection and stopped going. Or maybe she is still going to therapy, but it doesn't feel helpful because the therapist just listens to her "vent" and doesn't provide enough helpful feedback—or because the therapist provides too much feedback and doesn't allow her to express her feelings enough. Or maybe she loves the therapy and finds it incredibly helpful in the moment, but 6 months later nothing in her life has changed, and her PHQ-9 score remains stubbornly where it had been before she started treatment.

In other words, finding the right therapist for your patient is easier said than done. Prescribing psychotherapy is not like prescribing an antibiotic. It is not something you can simply arrange for a patient to do. There are many reasons for this—including a lack of available therapists relative to the need for them and systemic factors that make channels between primary care practices and psychotherapy practices difficult to maintain—but one thing that makes psychotherapy almost entirely beyond your control to arrange is that it is, at least in the way it is traditionally practiced, fundamentally a *relationship* between human beings.

For psychotherapy to work, the patient and the therapist need to form a genuine personal bond with each other [1]. This bond forms the basis of a *therapeutic alliance* through which the patient (or "client," depending on the discipline of the therapist) can come to expect empathy and expertise from the therapist while beginning to consider new ways of thinking about and interacting with the world around them. The therapeutic alliance alone is probably not sufficient for bringing most patients into a remission from their depression, but it is a foundation upon which therapy modalities are almost universally built. If it is not strong enough, the whole enterprise is likely to collapse. Moreover, if it is toxic (which it can be), the results are likely to be disastrous (Fig. 5.1).

Even if we were put aside the problem of interpersonal chemistry for a moment, finding any therapist at all who is able and willing to see new clients can also be extraordinarily difficult. To understand why, it may help to think about this from the perspective of a therapist (Fig. 5.2). The default therapy schedule in traditional settings involves 1 hour per week of direct clinical contact. The number of sessions needed is not usually defined, and many patients remain in treatment with the same therapist for years, or even decades. These parameters essentially limit the maximum number of clients that a typical therapist can actively work with at any given time (i.e., up to 40 in a 40-hour work week), although in practice this panel size can vary along with the true frequency of sessions for each client (which might be

Even though psychotherapy is not a medical or surgical intervention, it is not a treatment that is entirely without risk. Not everything that happens in a therapist's office is helpful to the patient, and not all patients come out happier for having done it.

An obvious instance of how psychotherapy can be harmful is "conversion therapy," in which a purported counselor attempts to change a client's sexual orientation through techniques that would not be widely accepted by the scientific community as "psychotherapy" but are nonetheless advertised as such. It is well established that attempts to change sexual orientation through therapy are associated with worse short-term and long-term outcomes than no treatment at all, and yet some practitioners continue to offer this.

Even mainstream psychotherapy treatments can go awry. For example, a study conducted during the late 20th century found that up to 10% of male therapists admitted to having romantic contact with their clients (which is not appropriate under any circumstances) highlighting how vulnerable patients seeking psychotherapy services are to being exploited.

Successful therapy requires that patients be able to trust their therapists. Although it is not realistic to expect that you as a referring provider will personally know and trust every therapist who provides care to one of your patients, it is a good idea to acknowledge that therapy is about a relationship and that there is no guarantee from the outset that this relationship will go well. If your patient doesn't feel comfortable with a particular therapist, this is likely not a result of his or her being a poor candidate for the work of psychotherapy, and it is OK to try shopping elsewhere.

Fig. 5.1 How psychotherapy can go wrong [2–4]

Fig. 5.2 A therapist's time is finite

There is some inescapable math about therapist availability that referring providers (and patients) should keep in mind: *the more personal time a therapist is dedicating to one patient, the less availability she or he has for other patients.* In other words, therapists who make themselves available to a higher volume of patients can give less personal attention to each one than therapists who maintain smaller panels can. You cannot have it both ways.

This is true of any clinician, including primary care providers! But many therapists (and some psychiatrists) practice independently and do not have the buffer of an interdisciplinary team to address patient needs beyond their face-to-face encounters. For them, all clinical care is direct clinical care.

multiple times per week or less often than once weekly), the rate of client turnover, and the hours that the therapist devotes each week to clinical care. Keep in mind that keeping clients in treatment longer is usually preferable from a business perspective and that many therapy practices are (by definition) small businesses.

Therapists who have recently opened up a new practice are likely to be receptive to new referrals, but demand for their services is high, and their schedules can fill up quickly. They will likely continue to have openings here and there according to client turnover, but they may also have their own referral networks or waiting lists that are beyond your reach as a primary care provider who is not already connected to them. For a specific therapist to have an opening at the right time for a specific patient can therefore require a great deal of luck (or in some cases, influence). A better bet is to build your own network, if you can.

So how do you do this?

The first step is to know who the players are and how their business models operate. Patients who are seeking care for the first time may not represent their needs accurately because they do not know the difference between a psychiatrist and a therapist, for example, and it may be necessary to educate them:

A *psychiatrist* is a physician who completed a residency program in psychiatry after finishing medical school. As with medicine or surgery, someone who trained in psychiatry may choose to specialize in one or more clinical areas, and these may or may not include a psychotherapy practice. Both supportive therapy and cognitive-behavioral therapy are core components of a psychiatrist's graduate medical education, but the rigor with which a psychiatrist must demonstrate excellence in these areas before graduating can vary by program [5]. It should therefore not be assumed that a psychiatrist has more experience as a therapist or a more sophisticated grasp of psychotherapy concepts than other types of clinicians who offer psychotherapy. It can almost always be assumed, on the other hand, that the cost per hour of hiring a psychiatrist for psychotherapy will be higher compared to most other disciplines.

A psychologist is someone who completed a doctoral training program in psychology. It is common to oversimplify the role of a psychologist on clinical teams by explaining that a psychologist performs psychotherapy while a psychiatrist can prescribe medication in addition to performing psychotherapy—which implies that a psychologist is basically like a psychiatrist but with fewer abilities. This is inaccurate, of course. Psychologists can develop a number of different skills in their graduate training programs and beyond, and these skills commonly include psychotherapy, which many psychiatrists can also do. Meanwhile, psychologists can practice other clinical skills that do not traditionally overlap with a psychiatrist's (e.g., certain kinds of psychological and neuropsychological testing) as well as important non-clinical skills that are more immediately relevant to scientific research, education, or business and entrepreneurship. Practically speaking, this means that many psychologists have full-time psychotherapy practices, and many do not. They may also be balancing their clinical work with other research and administrative obligations, meaning that the time they have time available to see new patients is highly variable.

A licensed mental health counselor (LMHC) or licensed professional counselor (LPC) is someone who completed a master's degree program in mental health counseling and has since gone on to meet the requirements for acquiring an independent license to practice mental health counseling in his or her state, which vary by location but generally involve some threshold of additional postgraduate training hours and passing a licensing examination. Licensed counselors are typically trained primarily for clinical psychotherapy services, and by the time they complete their requirements for certification they may have substantially more psychotherapy experience than many psychiatrists (and some psychologists). Like other kinds of health providers, they can also develop areas of sub-specialty expertise along the way. A counselor who spends most of his or her time treating substance use disorders may be less comfortable managing obsessive compulsive disorder, for example, and some counselors may offer only a specific range of modalities. Often, information about counselors' particular clinical areas will be posted on their websites or other online professional profiles.

Most primary care practices already work closely with social workers. However, similarly to many other disciplines, social work training is heterogeneous. Virtually all social workers have skills related to providing social and psychological support as well as crisis management, but some have more specialized training in the provision of direct mental health care services. Many social workers have full-time traditional psychotherapy practices, and others provide a combination of services that include but are not limited to psychotherapy in a variety of different settings. Social workers who are based in primary care clinics may or may not be formally trained as psychotherapists but nonetheless play a critical role in the assessment and management of patients with depression. They are often the first people called upon to provide support, counseling, and crisis management to patients even if this is not conducted under the auspices of a formal psychotherapy arrangement. They can also be an important liaison to long-term psychotherapy practices in the community.

Finally, nurses can provide psychotherapy services if they undergo postgraduate training for this, which typically involves advanced degrees and/or certification programs beyond a traditional nursing program. This training may be within the field of nursing (e.g., a nurse practitioner or clinical nurse specialist program), but some nurses also pursue degrees that are not directly related to their nursing backgrounds (e.g., a PhD in psychology). Either way, the training in psychotherapy that nurses receive is not significantly different from the training that other professional therapists receive. The most important difference between a nurse psychotherapist and any other psychotherapist is that he or she is also a nurse. In other words, their nursing backgrounds underlie their other skill sets and may inform their practice in certain ways just as other clinical backgrounds can inform practices in their own different ways.

It is unlikely that any one kind of training background is superior to any others when applied to providing psychotherapy to patients with depression in general. Instead, it is better to think about these disciplines as providing services that overlap in many respects but that can also include special expertise in certain areas that may be more or less relevant to some individual patients. Expertise in certain areas can also be developed in the years and decades that follow graduate training and certification, and the initials that come after the therapist's name can therefore be less informative than one might think. It is never a good idea to assume that a doctoral degree is a guarantee of a better psychotherapy experience.

It should not be surprising, then, that it is often difficult for psychiatrists to come to an agreement with insurance companies about paying substantially higher hourly rates for the psychotherapy services that they provide compared to clinicians with a master's degree. The issue of mental health parity in health care payments is deeper and more complicated than this, but one of its downstream consequences is that psychiatrists practicing outside of hospital systems are less likely to accept health insurance payments compared to other kinds of physicians [6, 7]. Therapists with other backgrounds may similarly accept only cash payments (since non-parity of reimbursement for mental health care services affects them as well), but their cash rates per hour may be within the budgets of more patients.

Beyond considering who is licensed to provide the psychotherapy treatments, it is also important to consider the treatment *modality*. Psychotherapy is not a single, unified practice that is consistently taught across all systems. Instead, it is a broad range of practices that apply different but often complementary strategies. It is also common for therapists to adopt an "eclectic" approach that incorporates techniques from multiple modalities into individualized treatments for each patient [8].

Combining modalities can be a good or bad thing. Administering a psychotherapy in its purest form, or according to the letter of a manual, ensures that it is done in accordance with what has actually been validated by research studies. On the other hand, there is something to be said for adaptability. Despite the variation in real-world practice, the majority of psychotherapy modalities align more closely with either of two dominant camps: psychodynamic/supportive therapy and cognitive behavioral therapy.

Psychodynamic Psychotherapy

Psychodynamic psychotherapy is the modern legacy of psychoanalysis and its founder, Dr. Sigmund Freud. In traditional psychoanalysis, a patient—or analysand—is instructed to lie on a couch facing away from the therapist—or analyst—and to start speaking about whatever comes to mind in that moment. The analyst then tries to interpret from this material and from any feelings that emerge in the room what kinds of unconscious desires and beliefs may be in conflict with the analysand's conscious identity and ultimately driving his or her psychopathology. Over an intensive regimen of four to five sessions per week that lasts many years, the analysand gradually gains enough insight about his or her unconscious mind that optimal psychological functioning can be restored.

True psychoanalysis can only be administered by a psychoanalyst. To become a psychoanalyst, psychotherapists must undergo years, or even decades, of intensive psychoanalytic training after they have already completed their initial licensures. This training involves classwork, providing psychoanalysis under the supervision of a training analyst, and personally undergoing psychoanalytic therapy. It is extremely time-consuming and expensive. Meanwhile, a devotion to research is not deeply embedded in the culture of psychoanalysis, and a solid basis of scientific evidence to support its efficacy or the validity of its core principles is lacking [9].

In other words, psychoanalysis in its traditional form does not fit neatly into the principles of value-based health care.

Modern psychodynamic therapy is much more practical. It adapts the principals of psychoanalysis to a schedule that is more manageable for most therapists and patients. In psychodynamic therapy, the therapist tries to help patients understand the ways in which their unconscious minds are affecting their lives, and then to support them as they try to change bad habits in response to this new insight [10]. In any particular treatment (or in any particular moment in the therapy), the therapist may be primarily focused on trying to provide support to the patient, or she or he may be more focused on trying to improve insight by uncovering unconscious material. Therapies that are more insight-oriented are commonly referred to as "insight-oriented therapies," whereas those that are more focused on supporting the patient are referred to as "supportive therapies." However, this is a false dichotomy. All psychodynamic therapies, by definition, are both insight-oriented and supportive, and whether or not a therapist skews to one set of techniques or another is only a matter of the patient's needs and abilities, the therapist's clinical decisions, and timing [10].

Psychodynamic therapy is effective for depression [1, 11, 12]. However, because individual psychodynamic treatments vary so widely in terms of content, the strength of the therapeutic alliance, and the duration, it is still somewhat difficult to study methodically. The desired outcomes from psychodynamic therapy are also likely to be more intangible than simply to "relieve depression" or another diagnosis-related symptom. Instead, many patients who undergo psychodynamic psychotherapy identify goals such as leading more productive lives or improving their relationships, and these are difficult to capture in measurements. Partly for these reasons, psychodynamic psychotherapy also does not fit neatly into the concept of a value-based health care system, and many psychodynamic therapists practice their crafts outside of traditional hospital systems.

Cognitive Behavioral Therapy

Cognitive behavioral therapy, or CBT, takes the opposite approach. It is structured (often following a manual), symptom-focused, and time-limited. It involves identifying and challenging unhelpful negative thoughts and then assigning homework exercises that are designed to reinforce more balanced and realistic beliefs or constructive reactions to stress [13]. Over time, individuals who have successfully undergone CBT see a measurable improvement in their target symptoms (depression, anxiety, panic attacks, etc.), and there is an enormous body of research to support its use [13, 14]. In addition to clinical research, neuroimaging studies have shown that structural and functional changes can occur in patients' brains as a response to CBT, further underscoring that it gets measurable results [15, 16]. In a way, the effects of CBT on brain structure and functioning can be compared to the effects of physical therapy on muscle structure and functioning: as the body adapts to using certain abilities more frequently and in a wider range of settings, those abilities are strengthened.

Given its time-limited nature, attention to specific and commonly reported symptoms, reliance on standardized protocols, and solid foundation in research, CBT embodies the spirt of value-based healthcare and has been widely embraced by hospital systems. Prescribers of CBT—in theory—can have a fairly good idea of both what the therapy should entail (i.e., the manual) and what it will cost (i.e., how

Fig. 5.3 Behavioral
activation therapy [19]

> *Behavioral activation* refers to a specific kind of
> homework assignment that is used in CBT for
> depression. In behavioral activation, the
> therapist guides the patient in scheduling
> activities throughout the week that promote
> feelings of enjoyment and mastery. It is highly
> effective both on its own and as a component of
> a more comprehensive treatment.
>
> Behavioral activation can also be successful
> when it is administered by clinical team
> members who are not formally trained in
> psychotherapy or even through technology-
> based platforms. It commonly serves as the
> backbone of programs that seek to extend the
> benefits of CBT to patients who would
> otherwise not have access to a traditional
> therapist.

many sessions) from the outset and can expect that its target outcomes will be immediately relevant to the diagnosed condition.

Despite CBT's advantages for interfacing with medical systems, referring to CBT is not a panacea. The supply of therapists who can reliably provide CBT is low relative to the need [14, 17], and not all therapists who advertise proficiency in CBT necessarily follow the treatment manuals faithfully [18]. Meanwhile, not all patients can relate to this treatment or are able and willing to follow through with the home-work exercises that are critical for its success.

In response to these treatment gaps, many program developers and entrepreneurs have adapted CBT to protocols that do not rely on a large time commitment from fully trained therapists. These adaptations include group therapies, simplifying or shortening the treatment itself (e.g., Behavioral Activation Therapy (Fig. 5.3), Problem-Solving Therapy), or delivering part or all of the therapy through a web-based platform [17, 19–23]. All of these adaptations can be effective, but they require different trade-offs and may ultimately look very different from what patients may have expected when they first agreed to try psychotherapy.

You can hopefully see now that a functional network for therapy referrals is not simply a Rolodex. A list of names and numbers to share with patients is nice to have, but the information it contains is likely to be incomplete and may go out of date more quickly than you can maintain it. That said, it is not a terrible starting point. Several therapist registries exist that cover a wide range of service needs and are easily accessible to you and your patients. If you have no other resources at hand, consider the following, along with their pearls and pitfalls:

Advising patients to call their insurance providers directly and ask for a list of therapists within their insurance networks is a common reasonable first step. In theory, seeking therapy within an insurance network ensures that it will be covered by the patient's plan and reduces the likelihood of surprise bills later on. In practice, this does not always work out. Calling an insurance company in the first place can be time-consuming, and the list of therapists that the patient eventually receives from the company may be out of date or inaccurate [24]. In other words, receiving a list of in-network therapists from an insurance company is unfortunately not a guarantee that the therapists on the list are currently in network or that the services they provide will be covered. Calling these therapists may also prove to be time-consuming in and of itself, and they may not be available to see new clients even if they can be reached. This process is understandably frustrating for many patients, but it works for some.

The website www.psychologytoday.com contains a therapist directory that can be used to search a large database of therapists who practice within a specified geographic area and have registered their profiles on the site. As with many other kinds of social media profiles, each therapist profile includes a photo, an autobiographical statement, a list of insurance plans accepted and areas of expertise, and the therapist's contact information. Therapists use this site as a form of advertising, and the information that they post in their profiles can be out of date or misleading at times (again, similarly to other kinds of social media). A statement on the profile that a therapist accepts payments from any particular insurance company can also carry multiple meanings and should not be taken at face value. This may mean that the insurance provider simply pays for the treatment minus a co-pay and/or a deductible, or it may mean that the insurance provider pays less than the full cost of treatment and that it is the patient's responsibility to cover the balance, however much that is. It could also mean that the patient has to pay for the full cost of the treatment up front but that the therapist will provide an invoice for the patient to submit to the insurance company for reimbursement while accepting the risk that this request for payment will be denied or stalled for any multitude of reasons. It is therefore critical for patients to ask for a complete explanation of how payment works from any prospective therapists before treatment starts in order to avoid any surprise bills (this is true no matter how the therapist was found).

Many state chapters of the National Association of Social Workers (NASW) also maintain "therapy matcher" services on their websites. Although the usefulness of these services can vary by state (and some state chapters may not offer this service), searching here may be another good starting point for many patients and referring providers. Links to individual state chapter websites can be found at the national NASW website, www.socialworkers.org.

Patients who are looking specifically for CBT can also search for one by using the Association for Behavioral and Cognitive Therapies' (ACBT) therapist directory, which is located at www.abct.org. Therapists who have registered their practices on this site have demonstrated at least some commitment to being a part of the CBT community, and they are ostensibly advertising their services as CBT providers. However, being registered with the ACBT still does not guarantee that a therapist is truly an expert in CBT or practices CBT faithfully according to its manuals.

In addition to these freely available directories, patients who have not yet found a therapist should be aware of the many self-help resources that might be sufficient to address mild or limited symptoms or otherwise might help them to get a head start on a more formal treatment that may not start right away. The ACBT also maintains a list of self-help books that are adherent to CBT and have been formally recommended by the organization, and it can similarly be found at www.abct.org.

Several web-based programs and apps have also been developed both to treat depression directly and to treat symptoms that are related to depression, such as insomnia, often using approaches that are rooted in CBT. The optimal role of these kinds of programs (e.g., as an alternative to versus complementary to traditional treatment) has not yet been established, but they appear to be effective for at least some patients, and they are likely better than no treatment [25–27]. Consensus guidelines regarding which programs or apps are the most effective and/or safe— and therefore appropriate to recommend—are currently lacking [28]. However, some non-profit agencies have consolidated helpful information about specific digital tools that can be accessed by patients who are considering or are interested in learning more about these treatments. These include the Anxiety and Depression Association of American (http://www.adaa.org/finding-help/mobile-apps), the One Mind PsyberGuide (https://oneminepsyberguide.org/apps/), and the m-Health Index and Navigation Database (MIND) library (https://mindapps.org/Home).

Finally, as you begin to construct your personal referral network, it is often helpful to leverage the networks that may already exist around you. Hospital systems and local behavioral health clinics can consolidate their triage processes and pool therapist availability, matching prospective patients to a waiting list and/or a "next available" clinician rather than to an individual therapist's turnover rate, which can be more unpredictable. Many (but not all) larger systems also accept insurance payments, including from Medicare and Medicaid, in a straightforward way that more closely aligns with other medical practices. A disadvantage of hospital systems and large clinics is that they may have restrictions on the types of treatment that can be offered or on which patients are eligible for services. Their wait lists can also grow so long that they become prohibitive.

Your colleagues may also have referral networks that they are willing to share. If you have a personal or working relationship with any behavioral health providers (including any social workers in your practice), feel free to ask them to recommend a therapist for your patients. Even if they are not practicing psychotherapy themselves, it is likely they trained with people who offer this service, particularly if they trained locally. They have also likely interacted with therapists in the community and may have a better idea of which ones are available to see new patients. If you happen to work in a hospital or group practice, other primary care providers may also have their own personal lists.

Some of your patients can also find therapists on their own. While it would be a boundary violation to ask any of your patients to help you find a therapist for another patient, it is reasonable to acknowledge that you are interested to know about good therapists in the area and to ask for their therapist's name and contact information, particularly if your patient is getting a good outcome from the therapy. With your patient's permission, you can then reach out to the therapist directly and ask whether she or he would be receptive to new referrals.

This is important: as you collect more detailed information about local therapists from different sources over time, keep it written down! You do not need a literal

Rolodex, but a personal directory of therapists (and/or practices) with whom you have personally communicated or who have been vetted by someone you know is difficult to maintain by memory alone. A successful network matures over a time span of years—not weeks—in practice, and over time, you will continue to learn more about what works (and what doesn't) for your patients.

References

1. Cuijpers P, Reijnders M, Huibers MJH. The role of common factors in psychotherapy outcomes. Annu Rev Clin Psychol. 2019;15:207–31.
2. Ryan C, Toomey RB, Diaz RM, Russell ST. Parent-initiated sexual orientation change efforts with LGBT adolescents: implications for young adult mental health and adjustment. J Homosex. 2020;67:159073.
3. Carr M, Robinson GE. Fatal attraction: the ethical and clinical dilemma of patient-therapist sex. Can J Psychiatr. 1990;35:122–7.
4. Appelbaum PS, Jorgenson L. Psychotherapist-patient sexual contact after termination of treatment: an analysis and a proposal. Am J Psychiatry. 1991;148:1466–73.
5. Accreditation Council for Graduate Medical Education. ACGME program requirements for graduate medical education in psychiatry. Revised June 13, 2020. https://www.acgme.org/Portals/0/PFAssets/ProgramRequirements/400_Psychiatry_2020.pdf?ver=2020-06-19-123110-817. Accessed 6/8/21 at 2:00pm.
6. Busch SH, Ndumele CD, Loveridge CF, Kyanko KA. Patient characteristics and treatment patterns among psychiatrists who do not accept private insurance. Psychiatr Serv. 2019;70:35–9.
7. Bishop TF, Press MJ, Keyhani S, Pincus HA. Acceptance of insurance by psychiatrists and the implications for access to mental health care. JAMA Psychiat. 2014;71:176–81.
8. Benjamin LS. The arts, crafts, and sciences of psychotherapy. J Clin Psychol. 2015;71:1070–82.
9. Paris J. Is psychoanalysis still relevant to psychiatry? Can J Psychiatr. 2017;62:308–12.
10. Cabaniss DL, Cherry S, Douglass CJ, Swhartz A. Psychodynamic psychotherapy: a clinical manual. Hoboken, NJ: John Wiley & Sons; 2011.
11. Leichsenring F, Rabung S. Effectiveness of long-term psychodynamic psychotherapy: a meta-analysis. JAMA. 2008;200:1551–65.
12. Dragioti E, Karathanos V, Gerdle B, Evangelou E. Does psychotherapy work? An umbrella review of meta-analyses of randomized controlled trials. Acta Psychiatr Scand. 2017;136:236–46.
13. Beck JS. Cognitive therapy: basics and beyond. New York, NY: The Guilford Press; 1995.
14. Kooistra LC, Wiersma JE, Ruwaard J, et al. Cost and effectiveness of blended versus standard cognitive behavioral therapy for outpatients with depression in routine specialized mental health care: pilot randomized controlled trial. J Med Internet Res. 2019;21:e14261.
15. Porto PR, Oliveira L, Mari J, et al. Does cognitive behavioral therapy change the brain? A systematic review of neuroimaging in anxiety disorders. J Neuropsychiatry Clin Neurosci. 2009;21:114–25.
16. Lazaridou A, Kim J, Cahalan CM, et al. Effects of cognitive-behavioral therapy (CBT) on brain connectivity supporting catastrophizing in fibromyalgia. Clin J Pain. 2017;33:215–21.
17. Richards DA, Ekers D, McMillan D, et al. Cost and outcome of behavioural activation versus cognitive behavioural therapy for depression (COBRA): a randomized, controlled, non-inferiority trial. Lancet. 2016;27:871–80.
18. Shafran R, Clark DM, Fairburn CG, et al. Mind the gap: improving the dissemination of CBT. Behav Res Ther. 2009;47:902–9.
19. Cuipers P, Quero S, Dowrick C, Arroll B. Psychological treatment of depression in primary care: recent developments. Curr Psychiatry Rep. 2019;21:129.

20. Bell AC, D'Zurilla TJ. Problem-solving therapy for depression: a meta-analysis. Clin Psychol Rev. 2009;29:348–53.
21. Huntley AL, Araya R, Salisbury C. Group psychological therapies for depression in the community: systematic review and meta-analysis. Br J Psychiatry. 2012;200:184–90.
22. Davies EB, Morriss R, Glazebrook C. Computer-delivered and web-based interventions to improve depression, anxiety, and psychological well-being of university students: a systematic review and meta-analysis. J Med Internet Res. 2014;16:e130.
23. Venkatesan A, Rahimi L, Kaur M, Mosunic C. Digital cognitive behavior therapy intervention for depression and anxiety: retrospective study. JMIR Ment Health. 2020;26:e21304.
24. Blech B, West JC, Yang Z, et al. Availability of network psychiatrists among the largest health insurance carriers in Washington, D.C. Psychiatr Serv. 2017;68:962–5.
25. Torous J, Cerrato P, Halamaka J. Targeting depressive symptoms with technology. Mhealth. 2019;5:19.
26. Marcelle ET, Nolting L, Hinshaw SP, Aguilera A. Effectiveness of a multimodal digital psychotherapy platform for adult depression: a naturalistic feasibility study. JMIR Mhealth Uhealth. 2019:e10948.
27. Moshe I, Terhorst Y, Philippi P, et al. Digital interventions for the treatment of depression: a meta-analytic review. Psychol Bull. 2021;147:749–86.
28. Lagan S, Sandler L, Torous J. Evaluating evaluation frameworks: a scoping review of frameworks for assessing health apps. BMJ Open. 2021;11:e047001.

Chapter 6
Treatment Resistance and Advanced Therapies

Approximately one third of patients with depression do not respond adequately to antidepressant treatment, even if it is administered according to evidence-based guidelines [1]. Of course, the experience of going through an antidepressant treatment and having it not work can be discouraging for patients and health providers alike. Failing to achieve remission after two treatments is even more difficult. This is a commonly accepted definition of treatment resistance in depression: *a failure to respond to two different antidepressant medications* [2].

This definition of treatment-resistant depression typically assumes that the antidepressant medications were either administered for a full therapeutic trial (i.e., at the maximum therapeutic dose for at least 8 weeks) or were discontinued as a result of intolerable side effects. However, this definition is not universal, and several alternative criteria have been both published and used in research studies [2]. Coming up with a unified approach to understanding and overcoming treatment resistance in depression is therefore especially challenging, and in clinical settings, it is important to consider treatment resistant cases from a big picture perspective rather than a series of checkboxes [3].

Consider the following case:

Marco is a 43-year-old man with a single episode of moderate-severe major depressive disorder. When you first evaluated him for this condition six months ago, you prescribed sertraline 50 mg daily. However, it upset his stomach, and he discontinued it after two days as a result. When he returned to you three months later, you prescribed escitalopram 10 mg daily, and he took this for 5 days before discontinuing it due to a perception that it was causing sexual side effects. He read online that he now meets criteria for treatment resistant depression—he is technically correct—and he asks if he could try ketamine next.

This case highlights how different individual experiences can be when it comes to treatment resistance, or perceived treatment resistance. Even though Marco technically could be considered to have treatment resistant depression (or TRD) on the basis of failing to respond adequately to two antidepressant medication trials as a

© The Author(s), under exclusive license to Springer Nature Switzerland AG 2022
D. S. Kroll, *Caring for Patients with Depression in Primary Care*, https://doi.org/10.1007/978-3-031-08495-9_6

result of "intolerable" side effects, it should be clear that ketamine—an advanced treatment that will be discussed later in this chapter—is not the right next step. A more accurate term to describe Marco's condition is *pseudo-resistance* [2].

Pseudo-resistance in depression—i.e., a failure to respond to antidepressant medication trials that are not truly therapeutic—is not always easy to identify, however. Marco's experience with medication comes from recent memory and is well-documented. Consider a different, more challenging example:

Deborah is a 37-year-old woman who has felt depressed for most of her life, and you have provided care to her for the last 2 years. She has gone through periods lasting months at a time in which she did not get out of bed as a result of her symptoms, and there have been other periods of relative improvement during which she was able to maintain stable employment for years at a time. However, her depression has never fully gone away. Her previous primary care provider prescribed fluoxetine and bupropion. Although both of these medication trials were associated with brief periods of feeling a little better, the perceived benefits did not last with either, and she has not taken any medications for depression in several years. She does not remember her doses or how long she took them for, and because she did not discuss discontinuing them with her providers at the time, there is no documentation in her health records to clarify this further. You have tried to refer her to psychotherapy twice, but these referrals have not been successful so far. Meanwhile, she is now hesitant to try another medication because, as she says, "Medication doesn't work for me."

This second case can be interpreted in a number of different ways. In one version of the story, Deborah has tried two conventional antidepressant medications that have different mechanisms of action, and neither of these medications was effective. In other words, her depression has been resistant to two first-line treatments, and she may require a more advanced approach—or at least a different one. In another version of the story, we have no way of knowing whether either of these medication trials was therapeutic. They may have been discontinued at a dose that was too low to be effective, or they may not have been given enough time to exert their effects. We also cannot assume that Deborah is recalling her experience correctly or that she was even taking her medications as prescribed during the time she claimed to be taking them in the first place.

While it is never a good idea to assume that a patient like Deborah is describing pseudo-resistance, at this stage, it is more accurate to say that her previous *treatment plans* were not effective—as opposed to saying that the medications themselves did not work for her. What she currently needs is a more reliable treatment plan, which may or may not involve trying the same medications (or the same family of medications) again, ideally incorporating efforts to systematically measure and document both the treatment and its response using the measurement-based care framework described in Chap. 3 [2].

So—practically speaking—how does this affect the next treatment steps?

An important first step, as always, is to collect as much information as you can about the previous treatment [3]. Does the patient remember any additional details, or is there any other reliable information to be found about the previous trials? Were any factors present at the time of the original treatment that might have confounded the assessment and/or treatment response, such as an unusual stressor (e.g., bereavement, homelessness, domestic violence)? Also, are there any indications of a diagnosis that is less likely to respond to conventional antidepressant treatments such as bipolar disorder, a personality disorder, or a substance use disorder?

Once you have maximized the information available to you—however much that is—the next step is to *optimize* the use of first-line treatments [3]. If there is not a compelling reason to avoid this, such as significant indicators of bipolar risk or a truly bad response to previous treatment, returning to an algorithm of first-line treatments is still appropriate. This might mean re-trying a medication that seemed not to be effective the first time, or it may mean trying something new that is still within the pantheon of first-line treatments (see Chap. 3). This time, however, use measurement-based care to ensure that a full therapeutic trial is completed and that the patient's response to treatment is clearly assessed and documented. If all goes well, you may find that the patient's depression responds favorably to treatment after all and that no further treatment steps are required.

Or you may not. After (or during) the full therapeutic trial, you may discover that the treatment is not effective at all for the patient's depression, or a persistent side effect may legitimately make it impossible to complete the full course of it. Alternatively, the depression may partially respond but still fail to remit even after 8 weeks at a maximum therapeutic medication dose.

If this happens, three additional office-based treatment options should be considered for the next steps: *switching, augmentation, and combining antidepressants* [3].

Switching to a different agent should be considered if there is absolutely no therapeutic response to the first treatment after a full therapeutic trial. Although it is not a hard rule, switching between classes (e.g., from an SSRI to bupropion) may be more effective than switching to another agent within the same class (e.g., from one SSRI to another SSRI) [3]. Practical strategies for switching between antidepressant agents are described in Chap. 3.

"Augmentation" refers to adding a second medication that is not traditionally classified as an antidepressant or is not typically used on its own to treat depression [3]. Examples include buspirone, lithium, triiodothyronine (T3), stimulants, and second- or third-generation antipsychotic medications [3, 4]. It is not a universal expectation that primary care providers should become comfortable prescribing any or all of these adjunctive agents (with or without a consulting psychiatrist to help), but it is still important to be familiar with how they are used and what their potential (both desirable and undesirable) effects are.

Buspirone

Buspirone is a serotonin receptor partial agonist that is associated with anxiolytic effects and has an independent role in the treatment of generalized anxiety disorder [5]. Unlike some anxiolytics, its use is not associated with a high risk of dependence, and it can be used safely as part of a long-term treatment plan [5]. As an augmenting agent for depressive disorders, it is typically administered at a dose of between 15 and 60 mg/day, spread out over two or three divided doses [6]. It is not required that a patient have co-morbid anxiety to be a candidate for adjunctive treatment with buspirone. However, the evidence basis supporting the efficacy of adjunctive buspirone is weaker than it is for some other agents, including antipsychotic medications [7]. At the same time, its profile for risks and side effects is more benign [7].

Common side effects of buspirone include nausea and dizziness [8]. Rarely, movement disorders such as dyskinesia or Parkinsonism have also been reported [9]. There is some evidence to suggest that it may offset the sexual side effects from SSRIs and SNRIs [6, 8].

Lithium

In addition to its role in bipolar disorder, lithium can improve recovery from unipolar depression when it is used adjunctively with conventional antidepressant treatments [2, 3, 4, 6]. It is typically initiated at a low dose (300-600 mg/d) and titrated to effective blood levels, similarly to how it is used in bipolar disorder [6]. However, unlike in bipolar disorder, where the target blood level is typically between 0.6–1.2 mmol/L, the optimal concentration for treating unipolar depression is not well characterized [6]. It is therefore reasonable for a patient to remain at a dose associated with a blood level below 0.6 mmol/L if it is clinically effective, although the traditional upper limit of 1.2 mmol/L remains a matter of safety and should not be exceeded. Some guidelines in fact suggest that lower target ranges (0.4–0.8 mmol/L) are more appropriate for treating or preventing depressive phases in bipolar disorder, and this may hold true for other types of depression as well [10].

Advantages of lithium include a relatively robust evidence basis to support its efficacy compared to other adjunctive treatments, its independent association with anti-suicidal effects, and other neuroprotective effects (including a possible decreased risk of developing dementia) [2, 6, 10, 11]. However, prescribing lithium also comes with special risks and inconveniences.

Acute toxicity, which typically occurs at blood levels of 2.0 mmol/L or higher, is a medical emergency. Patients may present at first with mild symptoms, such as weakness, light-headedness, and tremor but may also develop mental status changes, hemodynamic changes, and organ dysfunction in more advanced cases [12]. While appropriate laboratory monitoring can significantly mitigate the risk of a patient's developing lithium toxicity, it is not failsafe. Any conditions that impact renal functioning or serum concentrations of renally excreted molecules, either acutely (e.g., dehydration) or gradually, can lead to fluctuations in lithium blood levels. Because renal toxicity and nephrogenic diabetes insipidus can both develop insidiously as a result of chronic lithium toxicity even at therapeutic doses, the risk of acute toxicity can also increase over time and particularly for geriatric patients [10, 12]. Patients

Table 6.1 Monitoring recommendations for adjunctive treatments [2, 10, 12–16]

Drug	Initiation	Maintenance
Lithium	BUN, Creatinine	Initial: Lithium level 5 days after dose adjustment until stable
	TSH	First year: Lithium level, BUN, Cr, TSH, ECG, calcium every 6 months
	Calcium	After: Lithium level, BUN, Cr, TSH, ECG, calcium ever 12 months
	Pregnancy test	
	ECG	
T3	TSH	Repeat as clinically indicated
Stimulants	Height, weight, blood pressure, pulse	Repeat as clinically indicated
Antipsychotics	Height, weight, BMI	Repeat BMI every 3 months
	Waist circumference	Repeat A1C, lipid panel after 4 months
	Blood pressure, pulse	Annually thereafter: A1C, lipid panel, waist circumference, AIMS
	CBC, including absolute neutrophil count	
	BMP	
	LFT	
	TSH	
	A1C or fasting glucose	
	Lipid panel	
	Pregnancy test	
	ECG	
	AIMS	

AIMS Abnormal Involuntary Movement Scale

should be advised to skip their lithium doses if acute dehydration is to be expected, such as during times of acute gastrointestinal illness or even planned activities that carry a high risk of dehydration (e.g., running a marathon, hiking in the desert, etc.).

Long-term toxic effects, including renal impairment, nephrogenic diabetes insipidus, and thyroid dysfunction, can also develop over time even if toxic blood levels are never reached [10, 12]. Many patients also experience uncomfortable side effects that are unrelated to toxicity (although many others tolerate lithium without difficulty). It can therefore be cumbersome to prescribe, and prescribing it requires careful attention to laboratory monitoring requirements (Table 6.1) [2, 11].

Triiodothyronine (T3)

Thyroid hormone supplementation can be helpful as an adjunctive treatment even in patients who are euthyroid [6]. The usual starting dose is 25 mcg daily, and it can be increased to 50 mcg after the first week if there is no clinical response [6]. T3 is easier to prescribe than lithium and does not require the same degree of laboratory monitoring, although thyroid functioning should be assessed before starting it. On the other hand, there is less evidence to support its use in this context compared that supporting the use of lithium [2].

Stimulants

Central nervous system stimulants, such as methylphenidate, are traditionally used in the treatment of attention deficit/hyperactivity disorder (ADHD) but can also be used to directly treat fatigue and/or cognitive dysfunction in other health conditions [17, 18]. Their role in the adjunctive treatment of treatment-resistant depression is not well understood, but it is sometimes used for this purpose [17]. Current evidence suggests that there does seem to be a benefit for some patients, particularly with methylphenidate, for both depression severity and fatigue [17]. This potential benefit should be balanced with the potential risks, however, which include insomnia, increased anxiety, other undesirable mood changes, increased blood pressure, increased heart rate, and appetite suppression [13]. Before considering a stimulant, prescribers should also be mindful of its abuse potential as well as other potentially treatable factors that might be further contributing to fatigue or cognitive dysfunction, including benzodiazepines and other sedating medications.

Antipsychotic Medications

Second-generation antipsychotic medications have a strong evidence basis to support their use in treatment resistant depression, but they come with important caveats about risks and adverse effects. Although relatively easy to prescribe compared to lithium (in that their dosing does not need to be titrated to blood levels, and the necessary laboratory tests can be done less frequently), they should be prescribed cautiously. It is also not recommended that they be used for symptomatic relief of conditions such as insomnia that can occur in the absence of psychiatric conditions, even though they may be perceived as helpful [19].

Possible side effects of antipsychotic medications include sedation, orthostatic hypotension, anticholinergic effects, hyperprolactinemia, QTc-prolongation, weight gain, and metabolic syndrome [14]. They can also be associated with neurological effects, including dystonia, extrapyramidal symptoms, and tardive dyskinesia (which typically develops several years into treatment) [14, 15]. Some individual agents are greater offenders than others when it comes to specific side effect categories. Aripiprazole, for example, is much less likely to cause weight gain and metabolic problems compared to olanzapine, quetiapine, and risperidone, but it is relatively more likely to cause akathisia, or pathological restlessness [14, 20].

Before starting an antipsychotic medication, it is important to conduct a baseline physical assessment that includes the patient's weight, waist circumference,

comprehensive laboratory studies, and an ECG [14, 15]. It is also important to eval-
uate for abnormal involuntary movements using a standardized assessment tool
such as the Abnormal Involuntary Movement Scale (AIMS), and to repeat this
assessment at least annually throughout the course of treatment. Tardive dyskinesia,
while not dangerous (and less likely to occur with second-generation agents compared to older antipsychotic medications such as haloperidol), can become permanent even after antipsychotics are discontinued and is a common subject of
malpractice lawsuits [21, 22]. It is critical to ensure that the patient understands the
potentially permanent nature of tardive dyskinesia at the outset of treatment, to document this clearly in the health record, and to document that it has been monitored
for at regular intervals using standardized assessments.

Barring any emergent indications such as psychotic features or mania, antipsychotic medications should be initiated at the lowest therapeutic dose and then
increased to efficacy (unless prohibited by side effects) at intervals of 2–4 weeks [15].

Aripiprazole 2–20 mg Daily Aripiprazole is often a first consideration due to its
relatively low risk of metabolic side effects and a higher level of evidence for treating depression compared to other agents in the class [23]. It can be dosed in the
morning or at nighttime.

Brexpiprazole 0.5–3 mg Daily Brexpiprazole is structurally very similar to aripiprazole and appears to have a similar therapeutic and side effect profile [23, 24].
Because it is a relatively new agent, long-term effects are not well known [23].

Quetiapine 150–300 mg Daily Quetiapine is strongly sedating, even at low doses,
due to its antihistamine effects and should be dosed at bedtime. Although it can be
helpful for insomnia at low doses (e.g., 25 mg), the dosing range that has been
shown to be most effective for depression is between 150 and 300 mg daily [23].

Olanzapine 3–12 mg Daily Olanzapine is only FDA-approved for depression as
part of a combination with fluoxetine, which is marketed as Symbyax [24]. It is
highly sedating and typically dosed at bedtime similarly to quetiapine. It comes
with an especially high risk of significant weight gain and other metabolic side
effects [14].

Risperidone 0.5–2 mg Daily Risperidone is not FDA-approved for depression but
has been shown to be effective for treatment resistant depression in some studies
[23]. It therefore should not be considered as an early choice for augmentation, but
it remains a reasonable off-label option if other treatment options are unavailable or
exhausted.

Finally, combining antidepressants—i.e., using two or more antidepressant medications together—is a reasonable alternative to augmentation, although it has not
been studied as extensively for the purpose of enhancing treatment response as augmenting has [3]. It is important to keep in mind that if the first antidepressant medication was associated with no meaningful clinical improvement, it should be

discontinued rather than added to. If two or more antidepressant medications are to be combined, they also should not be from the same class. Moreover, if multiple agents with serotonergic effects are to be combined, they should not be used together in high dosing ranges due to the risk of their combination leading to serotonin toxicity (see Chap. 4). For example, while pairing sertraline 200 mg daily with bupropion 300 mg daily is unlikely to result in serotonin toxicity, a combination of sertraline 200 mg with venlafaxine 225 mg daily carries a higher risk that may or may not be justifiable depending on clinical circumstances.

Non-office-Based Treatments

The appropriateness of prescribing any of the above office-based treatments through primary care (as opposed to referring to a specialist) will vary by setting and institution, as well as by each individual provider's training and experience with advanced psychiatric treatments, with or without the support of an integrated care psychiatrist. By contrast, the following treatment options typically should *not* be delivered through primary care. Nonetheless, primary care providers often still have a role in these treatments, particularly when they require medical clearance (such as ECT), and should be aware of what they entail and what to expect from them.

Stimulation Therapies

The term "neurostimulation" refers to the application of electrical or magnetic energy to specific targets within the brain in order to achieve a therapeutic response [25]. Of course, this sounds like a highly invasive process, and it certainly can be (see Neurosurgical Treatments, below). However, both electroconvulsive therapy (ECT) and repetitive transcranial magnetic stimulation (rTMS) are tried and true therapies that are highly effective for depression.

ECT is in fact associated with higher treatment response rates than any antidepressant medication, with up to 80% of patients experiencing a benefit, and it is considered to be the most cost-effective treatment available for treatment-resistant depression [2, 6, 25]. It is heavily underutilized, in part because of stigma and because of a widely held misconception that it can be used as a punishment rather than a treatment after the way it was portrayed in *One Flew Over the Cuckoo's Nest* [2]. The actual procedure involves the use of electricity to induce a controlled seizure under anesthesia. It is usually administered two or three times per week for a total of between six and twelve treatments [6].

Primary care providers may be asked to perform a pre-treatment evaluation, which includes a basic medical clearance for general anesthesia and identifying medical conditions that could be relevant for determining which specific procedures are chosen. There are no absolute contraindications to ECT [6]. However, ECT activates both sympathetic and parasympathetic responses and can acutely cause increases in heart rate, blood pressure, cardiac work, and intracranial pressure [6, 26]. This means that certain patients—those with heart disease, space-occupying intracranial lesions, or a recent cerebral hemorrhage—may have a higher risk associated with the procedure, although these increased risks can also be managed if they are identified in advance [6, 25, 26].

A baseline cognitive examination should also be established. ECT can be associated with both anterograde and retrograde amnesia, especially in older adults, although this usually resolves, if not shortly after treatment than over a period of months after the treatment is completed [6]. Certain medications, especially those that can prevent seizures from occurring (antiepileptic drugs, benzodiazepines), limit the effectiveness of ECT and may also need to be discontinued prior to starting treatment [6].

In addition to its role in treatment-resistant depression, ECT should be considered earlier in cases of very severe depression or when there are psychotic or catatonic features [6].

rTMS involves the application of a magnetic inductor coil to the scalp in order to deliver magnetic pulses to specific brain regions [25]. Unlike ECT, it does not require anesthesia, and the most common side effects are scalp pain and headache [6, 25]. It does not typically cause cognitive side effects [25]. However, its typical regimen of five treatments per week for at least 20 sessions might be prohibitively inconvenient for some [6, 25].

Referral for rTMS does not usually require the same degree of medical clearance that ECT does. Patients with seizure disorders are often considered ineligible for rTMS because it may cause seizures in some patients [25].

Other non-surgical stimulation therapies—including transcranial direct current stimulation (tDCS) and magnetic seizure therapy (MST)—may also have a benefit in depression but have not been studied as rigorously as ECT and rTMS and are not considered to be first-line [2, 25].

Neurosurgical Treatments

There may also be a role for the use of surgically implanted electrical devices in the treatment of severe and highly refractory depression, but due to their invasiveness, level of risk, and relatively small evidence bases, these treatments should only be considered if all other reasonable options have failed.

Vagus Nerve Stimulation (VNS) involves placing an implantable pulse generator under the skin of the chest wall and connecting this to the vagus nerve via an electrode [2, 25]. It is approved only as an adjunctive treatment [6, 27].

Individuals who have had a VNS device implanted commonly develop dyspnea, coughing, voice alterations, and neck discomfort [6, 25]. There is also some risk of developing an infection related to the surgical procedure [6]. Once the device has been implanted, affected patients should also be aware of how the device can impact MRI procedures and/or the functioning of any other implanted devices [6].

Deep brain stimulation (DBS) similarly involves placing an implantable pulse generator in the chest, but this is instead connected to electrodes placed in the brain [2, 25]. This technique has been used more widely to treat movement disorders (e.g., Parkinson disease) and obsessive-compulsive disorder [28]. It appears to have some benefit in treating depression compared to sham treatments as well, but adverse events are also common, and it is still considered to be experimental [25, 29].

Ketamine and Esketamine

A single infusion of intravenous ketamine given at a sub-anesthetic dose of 0.5 mg/kg has been shown to relieve the symptoms of depression, including suicidal ideation, within as little as 4 hours and with effects lasting for up to 1 week [4, 30–32]. The mechanism for this benefit is unknown, as ketamine has effects on multiple neurotransmitter systems in addition to N-methyl-D-aspartate (NMDA) [33]. Also unknown are the long-term safety and efficacy of this treatment, and the optimal indications for it [31, 34].

On the one hand, ketamine is a promising and exciting treatment that many patients have already benefited from. Side effects are typically mild and include transient elevations in blood pressure and heart rate, dissociation, drowsiness, and dizziness [32]. On the other hand, it is not risk-free, and the treatment setting is important. Even though sub-anesthetic doses are called for, the facility in which ketamine is being administered should be capable of monitoring cardiovascular and respiratory status, and it should be appropriately staffed and equipped to respond to any potential adverse events, including hemodynamic instability [34]. In other words, it should not be administered in a private psychiatry office, and patients to whom this treatment has been recommended by a specialist should be steered toward reputable, well-equipped health centers if they have not been already.

There is also some reason to be concerned about ketamine's potential as a drug of abuse and about the role that activation of opioid receptors may play in mediating its antidepressant effects. Co-administering naltrexone with ketamine—and thus blocking its opioid effects—has been shown to also block its antidepressant benefits, suggesting that its effectiveness as an antidepressant is at least in part mediated by opioid activity [35]. While this does not necessarily mean that the increasing availability of ketamine as a treatment for depression is likely lead to pitfalls that are similar to the opioid epidemic, it is an important reminder to be cautious and to acknowledge that the long-term effects of this treatment are not yet known. It should not be considered until other, more conventional treatments have been demonstrated to be ineffective.

An intranasal formulation of a ketamine enantiomer—esketamine—has similarly been shown to be effective for treatment-resistant depression and to have a similar acute side effect profile to IV ketamine [33, 36–38]. Although it is administered as a nasal spray rather than an infusion, it should still be dosed under clinical supervision in a reputable health care facility.

While most primary care providers have not been trained to provide advanced depression treatments—especially those that are procedure-based or involve novel therapies—on their own, it is important to be aware of what patients may experience when they seek these treatments under the care of specialists. It is also important to understand that not all cases of depression that appear treatment resistant at first glance require advanced therapies. Clinicians should not be in a rush to recommend advanced therapies if there is not a compelling indication to do so (e.g., catatonic features necessitating ECT) and if lower-risk treatment options have not been exhausted, including cognitive behavioral therapy [39]. As with any other specialty, patients with treatment refractory psychiatric disease may consult a number of different providers and receive different and sometimes conflicting opinions about what is best for them. If they do, they will likely rely on their primary care providers to provide a voice of reason amidst all that noise.

References

1. Fava M, Davidson KG. Definition and epidemiology of treatment-resistant depression. Psychiatr Clin N Am. 1996;19:179–200.
2. Voineskos D, Daskalakis JZ, Blumberger DM. Management of treatment-resistant depression: challenges and strategies. Neuropsychiatr Dis Treat. 2020;16:221–34.
3. Ionescu DF, Rosenbaum JF, Alpert JE. Pharmacological approaches to the challenge of treatment-resistant depression. Dialogues Clin Neurosci. 2015;17:111–26.
4. McIntyre RS, Filteau M, Martin L, et al. Treatment-resistant depression: definitions, review of the evidence, and algorithmic approach. J Affect Disord. 2014;156:1–7.
5. Rickels K. Buspirone in clinical practice. J Clin Psychiatry. 1990;51(Suppl):51–4.
6. American Psychiatric Association. Practice guideline for the treatment of patients with major depressive disorder. 3rd ed; 2010.
7. Davies P, Ijaz S, Williams CJ, et al. Pharmacological interventions for treatment-resistant depression in adults. Cochrane Database Syst Rev. 2019;2019:CD010557.
8. Garakani A, Murrough JW, Freire RC, et al. Pharmacotherapy of anxiety disorders: current and emerging treatment options. Front Psych. 2020;11:595584.
9. Rissardo JP, Caprara ALF. Buspirone-associated movement disorders: a literature review. Prague Med Rep. 2020;121:5–24.
10. Malhi GS, Gessler D, Outhred T. The use of lithium for the treatment of bipolar disorder: recommendations from clinical practice guidelines. J Affect Disord. 2017;217:266–80.
11. Post RM. The new news about lithium: an underutilized treatment in the United States. Neuropsychopharmacology. 2018;43:1174–9.
12. MacLeod-Glover N, Chuang R. Chronic lithium toxicity: considerations and systems analysis. Can Fam Physician. 2020;66:258–61.
13. Thapar A, Cooper M. Attention deficit hyperactivity disorder. Lancet. 2016;387:1240–50.

14. Viron M, Baggett T, Hill M, Freudenreich O. Schizophrenia for primary care providers: how to contribute to the care of a vulnerable patient population. Am J Med. 2012;125:223–330.
15. American Psychiatric Association. The American Psychiatric Association practice guidelines for the treatment of patients with schizophrenia. 3rd ed. Washington, DC: American Psychiatric Association; 2021.
16. American Psychiatric Association. Practice guideline for the treatment of patients with bipolar disorder. 2nd ed. Washington, DC: American Psychiatric Association; 2010.
17. Bahji A, Mesbah-Oskui L. Comparative efficacy of stimulant-type medications for depression: a systematic review and network meta-analysis. J Affect Disord. 2021;292:416–23.
18. Andrew BN, Guan NC, Jaafar N. The use of methylphenidate for physical and psychological symptoms in cancer patients: a review. Curr Drug Targets. 2018;19:877–87.
19. Anderson SL, Vande Griend JP. Quetiapine for insomnia: a review of the literature. Am J Health Syst Pharm. 2014;71:394–402.
20. Preda A, Shapiro BB. A safety evaluation of aripiprazole in the treatment of schizophrenia. Expert Opin Drug Saf. 2020;19:1529–38.
21. Carbon M, Hsieh C, Kane JM, Correll CU. Tardive dyskinesia prevalence in the period of second-generation antipsychotic use: a meta-analysis. J Clin Psychiatry. 2017;78:e264-78.
22. Shriqui CL, Bradwejn J, Jones BD. Tardive dyskinesia: legal and preventive aspects. Can J Psychiatr. 1990;35:576–80.
23. Cantù F, Ciappolino V, Enrico P, et al. Augmentation with atypical antipsychotics for treatment-resistant depression. J Affect Disord. 2021;280(Pt A):45–53.
24. Fornaro M, Fusco A, Anastasia A, et al. Brexpiprazole for treatment-resistant major depressive disorder. Expert Opin Pharmacother. 2019;20:1925–33.
25. Milev RV, Giacobbe P, Kennedy SH, et al. Canadian network for mood and anxiety treatments (CANMAT) 2016 clinical guidelines for the management of adults with major depressive disorder: section 4. neurostimulation treatments. Can J Psychiatr. 2016;61:561–75.
26. Hermida AP, Mohsin M, Marques Pinheiro AP, et al. Cardiovascular side effects of electroconvulsive therapy and their management. J ECT. 2021; https://doi.org/10.1097/YCT.0000000000000802.
27. Bottomley JM, LeReun C, Diamantopoulos A, et al. Vagus nerve stimulation (VNS) therapy in patients with treatment resistant depression: a systematic review and meta-analysis. Compr Psychiatry. 2019;98:152156.
28. Krauss JK, Lipsman N, Azizi T, et al. Technology of deep brain stimulation: current status and future directions. Nat Rev Neurol. 2021;17:75–87.
29. Kisely S, Li A, Warren N, Siskind D. A systematic review and meta-analysis of deep brain stimulation for depression. Depress Anxiety. 2018;35:468–80.
30. Phillips JL, Norris S, Talbot J, et al. Single, repeated, and maintenance ketamine infusions for treatment-resistant depression: a randomized controlled trial. Am J Psychiatry. 2019;176:401–9.
31. Marcantoni WS, Akoumba BS, Wassef M, et al. A systematic review and meta-analysis of the efficacy of intravenous ketamine infusion for treatment resistant depression: January 2009-January 2019. J Affect Disord. 2020;277:831–41.
32. DeWilde KE, Levitch CF, Murrough JW, et al. The promise of ketamine for treatment-resistant depression: current evidence and future directions. Ann N Y Acad Sci. 2015;1345:47–58.
33. Swainson J, Thomas RK, Archer S, et al. Esketamine for treatment resistant depression. Expert Rev Neurother. 2019;19:899–911.
34. Sanacora G, Frye MA, McDonald W, et al. A consensus statement on the use of ketamine in the treatment of mood disorders. JAMA Psychiat. 2017;74:399–405.
35. Williams NR, Heifets BD, Blasey C, et al. Attenuation of antidepressant effects of ketamine by opioid receptor antagonism. Am J Psychiatry. 2018;175:1205–15.
36. Popova V, Daly EJ, Trivedi M, et al. Efficacy and safety of flexibly dosed esketamine nasal spray combined with a newly initiated oral antidepressant in treatment-resistant depression: a randomized double-blind active-controlled study. Am J Psychiatry. 2019;176:428–38.

37. Daly EJ, Singh JB, Fedgchin M, et al. Efficacy and safety of intranasal esketamine adjunctive to oral antidepressant therapy in treatment-resistant depression. JAMA Psychiat. 2018;75:139–48.
38. Daly EJ, Trivedi MH, Janik A, et al. Efficacy of esketamine nasal spray plus oral antidepressant treatment for relapse prevention in patients with treatment-resistant depression: a randomized clinical trial. JAMA Psychiat. 2019;
39. Li JM, Zhang Y, Su W, et al. Cognitive behavioral therapy for treatment-resistant depression: a systematic review and meta-analysis. Psychiatry Res. 2018;268:243–50.

Chapter 7
Managing Suicide Risk

Suicide is the tenth leading cause of death in the United States [1, 2]. In 2019, which is the most recent year for which global suicide estimates have been published by the World Health Organization at the time of this writing, more than 700,000 people died from suicide—more than 1% of all deaths worldwide [3]. More people died from suicide that year than from breast cancer, HIV/AIDS, malaria, or war [3].

Yet suicide is unique among causes of death in that the victim of a suicide has, by definition, chosen to die. Possibly because it is so closely linked to a conscious decision [4], bystanders in the wake of a suicide (including family, friends, and, of course, clinicians who cared for the decedent) are often left with a special combination of helplessness—since humans have free will, after all—and guilt. It is hard not to believe that something could have been done or said to prevent it from happening, *if only we had known.*

While it is conceivably true that doing or saying the right thing at exactly the right point in time can save somebody's life, this is, of course, an oversimplification. Nearly half of all people who die from suicide have visited their primary care providers in the month prior to their deaths [5], so it is natural to think that primary care providers should do something about it. And you should! But doing your due diligence—and more—does not mean taking on the sole responsibility for the outcome. Effective suicide prevention does not mean that you can prevent every single suicide from happening. This would be difficult even if you had both a crystal ball (that actually works) and a major military power at your disposal, and so far, no evidence-based protocols for suicide prevention have demonstrated that even these tools can be effective 100% of the time.

This is important to be frank about: *you cannot stop suicide.* That cannot be an appropriate goal because it is impossible to achieve. It is essential to shift the frame, or else we are guaranteed to fail.

A health care provider's job has never been to control what patients do or how they die. This can be said about any medical condition or behavior, and suicide is no exception, even if many of us cannot shake the illusion that it is. Instead, *a health*

© The Author(s), under exclusive license to Springer Nature
Switzerland AG 2022
D. S. Kroll, *Caring for Patients with Depression in Primary Care,*
https://doi.org/10.1007/978-3-031-08495-9_7

care provider's job is to follow evidence-based practices with regard to screening for, assessing, and managing suicide risk and any associated health conditions. It is also to create a treatment environment in which patients who are grappling with a desire to end their lives have an opportunity to identify themselves as such if they choose to and to access medical or social resources that can either directly mitigate their risk or repair the underlying factors that may be driving them to despair.

Consider the following case:

KG is a 68-year-old white man with a history of chronic, treatment-resistant depression and a family history of suicide by way of his grandmother. You have strongly recommended that he accept a referral to a psychiatrist and therapist multiple times over the years, but he refuses. He has worked with different psychiatrists and therapists on and off for decades and tried every medication that you can think of in addition to ECT, and nothing has ever resulted in any meaningful symptom relief. He simply does not see the point in pursuing treatment any longer, and even his last psychiatrist told him (this was fifteen years ago) that there was nothing left to gain from further treatment. So instead, he comes to you every few months, fills out a PHQ-9 (which always produces a score of 27), and rejects any kind of help you try to offer.

He has been fantasizing about suicide for least the last 40 years, and his fantasy involves driving to a remote place in the woods and shooting himself. He owns a gun, and he is fully capable of carrying out this plan if he ever chooses to do so. But so far, he hasn't. He has never made any attempt—or even taken any steps in preparation for an attempt—to end his life. He has been psychiatrically hospitalized multiple times, but this has also never been helpful.

It may seem like there is not a lot you can do about this problem, but in fact there is—and not just sending KG to the hospital (again) simply for a lack of any better options. Sending KG to the hospital *might* be appropriate, but you have not yet been given enough information to make that determination. You are going to need more.

As an overview, it may be helpful to start by breaking down this process into three steps: **screening**, **assessment**, and **management**. They are different from each other, but they will all fit together into a cohesive strategy before the end of this chapter.

Screening, in this case (as in any other), means identifying the patients who may be at risk of suicide from among all the patients who could potentially be at risk (i.e., all patients). That statement may be obvious, but the reason I define screening here is to distinguish it from *assessment*, even though these two actions share a few overlapping parts. The primary purpose of a screen is to start with a general population and determine who among that group might require further attention. No existing screening protocol for suicide risk has been shown to be 100% sensitive, and therefore you will not be successful in identifying every single patient who is at risk no matter what you do, but using an evidence-based method is a good place to start (more on this later).

Screening does not have any clinical value for a patient like KG because he has already identified himself as someone who may be at risk of suicide. You do not need to administer a screening tool to know that KG requires further assessment.

However, amplifying the signal that KG is suicidal is not the purpose of a screen. The purpose of a screen is to systematically ensure that all patients—who may or may not be as vocal about the despair that they are feeling as KG is—receive the same inquiry into their risk regardless of what their clinicians expect the screen to show.

It is important to acknowledge also that screening alone has not been shown to lower suicide rates and should not be the cornerstone of anyone's strategy [6]. It is only a starting point.

Assessment involves gathering more information and determining the level of risk. The gold standard for this process is to conduct a psychiatric diagnostic assessment [7], but this does not mean that every patient with suicidal ideation needs to be evaluated by a *psychiatrist*. Instead, it means that the patient should be asked additional questions about their thoughts on suicide and evaluated for the presence of a psychiatric illness as well as any pertinent risk factors and protective factors. Gathering this information will allow you to comprehensively assess the patient and ascertain what the most appropriate next steps will be.

As part of this assessment, it is important to ask about the patient's suicidal ideation in detail, including whether the patient has developed a suicide plan and whether she or he has any intention of acting on this plan and/or the means to do so. This includes asking about firearms. Asking about this and acknowledging that access to firearms is an important modifiable risk factor for suicide death is not the same as saying that patients who have ever thought about suicide should not be allowed to own guns—any more than advising other patients about wearing seatbelts would imply that they should not be allowed to drive cars. However, some patients may feel challenged when their providers initiate a discussion about firearm safety, and a range of responses to this line of questioning should be expected. More information about why this is important is contained in Fig. 7.1.

Although many individuals consider suicide for long periods of time--sometimes years--acute suicidal intent usually lasts for less than one hour at a time. This is why restricting access to means is so important in suicide prevention efforts. Although individuals who are truly determined to end their lives will often find a way to do so no matter who or what tries to stop them, simply slowing the process down can have a significant impact.

Many of us associate the idea of "restricting access to means" with controlling access to firearms, but this association exists in the United States mainly because firearms are relatively available in many states and are involved in approximately 50% of American suicide deaths. However, experience in other countries shows that this concept is applicable to other suicide methods, too.

For example, before the 1950s, approximatley 1/3 of all suicide deaths in England were associated with gas poisoning. At the time, putting one's head in the oven was often seen as the most expedient and immediately accessible method for dying by suicide, and so it was popular (in a manner of speaking). When the country converted from poisonous charcoal gas to natural gas, which is safer, this option suddenly went away, and a significant drop in overall suicide rates was seen nationally.

In other countries, limiting access to pesticides or jumping sites can be similarly beneficial. Restricting access to means can signify different interventions in different places and for different patients

---

Fig. 7.1 Restricting access to means [7–11]

Table 7.1 Suicide risk factors [4, 12, 13]

Historical factors	Biological factors	Demographic factors	Psychological traits	Social factors	Psychiatric disorders
Previous suicide attempts	Genetic factors	Male gender	Anhedonia	Relationship conflicts	Mood disorders
Previous self-injury	Medical illness	White race	Impulsivity	Legal problems	Impulse control disorders
Family history of suicide		Native American race (in the United States)	Hopelessness	Access to means	Personality disorders
Childhood trauma		LGBTQ+ status	Perfectionism	Suicidal behavior in peers	Psychotic disorders
		Age (young adult or older adult)	Emotional reactivity		Substance use disorders

This step also includes taking a detailed history that identifies pertinent risk factors and protective factors. Risk factors, some of which are listed in Table 7.1, can be considered modifiable or non-modifiable (Table 7.1). A non-modifiable risk factor is a historical fact that predisposes a patient to a higher suicide risk but cannot be changed even with optimal treatment. Examples include a history of prior suicide attempts, a family history of suicide, and certain demographic factors. Modifiable risk factors are those that can potentially be improved with an intervention—e.g., major depressive disorder or access to weapons. Protective factors confer a lower suicide risk. Examples include spiritual or religious beliefs against suicide, strong psychosocial support, a patient's individual strengths, and identified reasons for living [7].

The purpose of sorting out the risk factors and protective factors is not to quantify the immediate suicide risk per se. Many of these factors can even carry a different meaning in different settings and populations—for example, associations between gender and suicide vary across countries, and associations between advanced age and suicide risk can change according to race (although the association between being a young adult and suicide holds true across demographic groups) [7]. Being married is typically considered a protective factor, but if the marriage is plagued by violence at home, it becomes a risk factor [7]. Meanwhile, the actual predictive validity of any individual risk factor is poor, especially for near-term risk [13, 14]. The goal of sorting through this information is instead to better characterize the realities that each patient is dealing with, for better or worse, and to make a distinction between which factors could become potential treatment targets (i.e., modifiable factors)—and which cannot.

Finally, the assessment should also include a general psychiatric history and an inquiry into current symptoms as well as substance use habits. Insomnia in particular should be noted if it is present because insomnia is acutely associated with suicide risk and is also rapidly treatable in many cases [7, 15]. An accurate psychiatric diagnosis will also inform an optimal treatment plan; however, it is important to keep in mind that suicide is not inextricably linked to having a psychiatric disorder, and many individuals who do not have psychiatric disorders still die from suicide [16].

It is also important to acknowledge that not all patients will be completely candid with their providers about information that pertains to mental health and suicide, and patients can also change their minds about suicide after being assessed [17]. These are unavoidable facts of dealing with human beings, especially around a topic that is as highly stigmatized as suicide is. However, for most patients in primary care, a suicide risk assessment is a longitudinal process in which relevant information accumulates over time and comes in from multiple sources. Especially when the stakes are acutely high, it is often a good idea to solicit information from collateral sources, such as family members or other health providers, whenever possible [7]. Ideally, this should happen with the patient's full participation and consent. However, even if the patient does not consent to your sharing information with other people, collateral information may still become available beyond the patient's control or the bounds of HIPAA (e.g., through unsolicited outreach by family members or through information that is already documented in the health record), and it is still appropriate to consider that information when it is presented.

Management refers to developing and implementing a strategy for optimally treating the underlying psychiatric illness (if present), addressing modifiable risk factors to the extent that this is practical, and mobilizing protective factors when this is possible. Sometimes, this also requires taking steps to contain the risk of suicide when it is acutely and immediately high.

Determining the right level of care for a patient with suicidal ideation is critical, but it also requires an act of faith. This is, of course, the step for which that crystal ball would come in the handiest. Patients who are immediately on the verge of ending their lives—i.e., those who are currently within the one-hour window of peak suicidal activity or are likely to arrive there before the next business day [8]—are likely to require a *containment* strategy. Containment—i.e., taking steps to directly limit someone's freedom, usually by pursuing admission to a locked psychiatric ward or sometimes even applying a restraint—is not failsafe, however. It carries significant risks of its own—including stripping patients of certain rights, potentially injuring them, and the inviting the possibility that they may still find a way to kill themselves even in a setting that is designed to protect them from that very outcome [18]. In some cases, applying a coercive treatment can also disrupt the clinical relationship and discourage patients from future treatment engagement [19].

Striking the right balance between these two highly problematic choices—restrict a patient's freedom (in accordance with state laws and other local ordinances) or potentially miss an opportunity to save a life—is extraordinarily hard to do. It is all the more difficult because, unfortunately, a working crystal ball has not yet been invented at the time of this writing. But remember that a health provider's job is not to prevent 100% of suicides, but rather to make the best clinical decision with the information that is available or can reasonably be made available. I will even take this one step further: *if you are providing the best possible care, you are going to miss acute suicide risk in some cases.*

In other medical conditions, the concept of the "threshold approach" to clinical decisions is perhaps more readily understood and accepted [20]. There is some likelihood of harm associated with an intervention, and there is another likelihood of harm associated with withholding that intervention. If the treatment or diagnostic intervention is less likely to cause harm than the untreated or undiagnosed condition, go forward. But if the risk/benefit ratio is reversed, it is better to forego that intervention [20].

Notice that this is not the same as saying that if the intervention will cause more harm than good, do not proceed. None of us knows in advance what the outcome of any intervention (or lack thereof) will be for an individual patient. We can only know the likelihood—and even this can have an uncomfortably wide margin of error.

Consider the predicament of an emergency physician and a patient with a possible pulmonary embolism (PE) [21, 22]. Several clinical and laboratory criteria exist to help support emergency department providers in determining whether a PE is present, but ultimately, a CT scan is definitive. In other words, if the emergency provider orders a CT scan on every single patient who *might* have a PE, she or he will not miss PEs. A CT scan is not benign, however. It exposes the patient to ionizing radiation, slows down treatment, comes with a high cost, and may ultimately delay treatment for other patients who are waiting for their turn in the scanner [21]. A responsible emergency department provider therefore has to balance these risks and does *not* send every patient for a CT scan. Doing so would be unnecessary for a high number of patients and cause more harm overall. It turns out that when the emergency physician is practicing the best possible evidence-based medicine, the miss rate for PEs is approximately 2% [21, 22]. Not zero.

There is much about our culture that makes us feel that we should be held to a higher standard when it comes to suicide. And of course, we should—*in a perfect world*. But evidence-based medicine does not support this standard yet. The best we can do as clinicians is to rely on the best evidence-based practices that are currently available and to offer treatment for the medical, psychiatric, and psychosocial conditions that underlie suicide risk.

There is still a lot that can be done to help reduce suicide risk that does not involve restraining patients or restricting their freedoms, and the vast majority of patients with suicidal ideation do not require hospitalization. The first, and arguably most important, intervention is to treat the underlying depression, or another psychiatric disorder, when it is present. Although not all psychiatric treatments have been demonstrated to reduce suicidal ideation and suicide risk directly, psychiatric conditions remain among the most important (and treatable) modifiable risk factors for suicide and should always be addressed as part of the treatment plan in cases where suicide risk is a consideration. Medical and psychological treatments that have been demonstrated to reduce suicide risk directly are listed in Table 7.2.

A process called "safety planning" can also be an effective tool. It is critical to distinguish "safety planning" from a "safety contract" or "contracting for safety," however, as these latter strategies are known *not* to be effective [7, 29]. To say that a patient has "contracted for safety" means that the patient has promised not to engage in suicidal behavior or to seek emergency services if she or he feels that suicidal behavior is imminent. However, contracting for safety is not associated with a reduced suicide risk, and even writing the words "contracted for safety" in the health record should be avoided, as this could insinuate that the "contract" was considered a factor in the suicide risk assessment (which it should not be).

Table 7.2 Treatments with efficacy in reducing suicide risk [7, 9, 23–28]

Medications
Lithium
Clozapine
Ketamine
Psychotherapies
Dialectical Behavioral Therapy (DBT)
Safety Planning Intervention (SPI)
Cognitive Therapy for Suicide Prevention (SP-SP)
Collaborative Assessment and Management of Suicidality (CAMS)
Attempted Suicide Short Intervention Program (ASSIP)
Other somatic treatments
Electroconvulsive Therapy (ECT)
Repetitive Transcranial Magnetic Stimulation (rTMS)

In safety planning, the clinician and patient collaborate to develop a "written, prioritized list of strategies and sources of support" that can be accessed in the event of an acute suicide crisis [30]. The components of a safety plan include identifying warning signs, applying coping strategies, restricting access to means, and accessing one's support network, which can include family, friends, and health care providers [30]. Training in the use of a safety plan is beyond the scope of this chapter, but resources are available online and can be accessed at https://suicidesafetyplan.com.

Whenever it is possible and practical to do so, it is a good idea to engage other team members and supportive family members or significant others in the process, as they can help to create a stronger support network and also facilitate risk mitigation steps, including the limiting of access to means when appropriate. Framing this process as a team approach rather than an individual treatment decision may also help to mitigate the tendency of some health providers to treat patients with suicide risk like a "hot potato"—i.e., to prioritize not being the last point of contact before a suicide occurs and rely excessively on risk containment rather than advancing the psychiatric treatment plan.

Finally, the documentation in the health record should describe the decision-making process in a way that is honest and candid. This should include any relevant information that was reviewed, whatever treatment or containment steps were taken or not, and any consultations or collaborations that took place [7]. A few examples of language that might be used in difficult scenarios are listed in Fig. 7.2.

For any of this to work, of course, it all needs to come together into a coherent protocol. Fortunately, when The Joint Commission (TJC) began mandating that all health care organizations accredited as hospitals in the United States begin following an evidence-based protocol for screening for and assessing suicide risk in 2019, it provided a pretty good set of instructions for how to do so [31]. Not all primary care providers are beholden to TJC's requirements because not all primary care providers are practicing in organizations that are accredited as hospitals. However, the standards that TJC has established are likely to be helpful no matter what setting you are in.

The requirements that were set by TJC as part of 2019's National Patient Safety Goal 15.01.01 are summarized in Table 7.3. They pertain specifically to

Chronic risk

Although this patient has a chronic baseline risk, and expressions of suicidal ideation do not necessarily indicate acute risk on their own, the symptoms that the patient presents with today are more severe than their baseline level, and his suicide risk is therefore acutely elevated and in need of further assessment (or immediate containment, etc.) Although this patient has multiple modifiable and non-modifiable risk factors for suicide and has a high baseline risk for dyingfrom suicide, there are no indications at this time that this risk is acutely elevated or that hospitalization or restraint is likely to mitigate this risk. Therefore, continuing outpatient treatment is more likely to be effective as a long-term plan.

Trauma history that limits the benefit of hospitalization or restraint

Although I am concerned about the ongoing risk of suicide that could occur in the outpatient setting even in the course of treatment, given this patient's trauma history and previous experiences in locked hospital settings, which were unhelpful, I do not think that pursuing any involuntary containment strategy has a favorable risk/benefit ratio in this case. I have significant concern that an involuntary treatment setting would exacerbate her symptoms and ultimately her overall suicide risk rather than provide relief, and at the gain of only a very short-term risk reduction, and therefore I think that continuing outpatient treatment remains the most likely strategy achieve the best possible outcome andoverall safety profile.

Concern for malingering

The patient's statements in this case are difficult to interpret because her stated suicidal intentions cannot be considered a reliable indicator of her actual suicide risk due to her history of making similar statements falsely and the ongoing potential for secondary gain. This does not necessarily mean that she does not have an acute suicide risk at this time, but rather that her statements regarding suicidal intentions do not historically correlate well with her true risk, and other risk indicators must be relied upon instead. At this time, a thorough examination and a review of her health records do not reveal any acute changes in her symptoms or circumstances that would suggest a change in her risk level compared with her baseline, nor do they reveal a treatment target that could be treated more effectively in a more restrictive setting. Conversely, repeatedly admitting her to the hospital--which has already been demonstrated to be ineffective in reducing either her symptoms or her stated suicide risk for any sustained period of time—may be doing more harm than good by directing her care to an incorrect and ineffective treatment setting rather than a potentially more sustainable outpatient treatment plan.

Fig. 7.2 Examples of documenting complex suicide risk assessments

Table 7.3 The Joint Commission's national patient safety goal 15.01.01: reduce the risk for suicide [31]

Element of performance	Requirement
1	The organization conducts an environmental risk assessment that identifies features in the physical environment that could be used to attempt suicide and takes necessary action to minimize risks
2[a]	**Screen all individuals served for suicidal ideation using a validated screening tool**
3[a]	**Use an evidence-based process to conduct a suicide risk assessment of individuals served who have screened positive for suicidal ideation. This assessment should directly ask about suicidal ideation, plan, intent, suicidal or self-injurious behaviors, risk factors, and protective factors**
4[a]	**Document the level of overall suicide risk and the plan to mitigate that risk**
5	Follow written policies and procedures addressing the care of individuals who have been identified at risk of suicide.
6	Follow written policies and procedures for counseling and follow-up care at discharge for individuals identified as at risk of suicide
7	Monitor implementation and effectiveness of policies and procedures for screening, assessment, and management of individuals at risk of suicide and take action as needed to improve compliance

[a]EPs that individual outpatient clinicians can be considered directly accountable are identified in bold

patients who have presented with a behavioral health problem as the primary reason for their care and are oriented chiefly toward hospital systems. A primary care provider practicing in the outpatient setting does not need to ensure that her examination room is "ligature resistant" in the same way that emergency departments need to be, for example (i.e., it is not required that the room be devoid of any protrusions—such as a drawer handle—that might conceivably be used to tie a bedsheet around, etc.) [31]. These requirements also apply only to patients who are presenting with a chief complaint related to behavioral health symptoms or a behavioral health condition. This means that patients who are presenting with a primary medical condition (e.g., ankle pain, diabetes care) do not need to receive a suicide screening protocol according to TJC, whereas patients with any behavioral health chief complaint (including depression, anxiety, substance use, etc.) do. If a patient initially presents with a chief complaint related to a general medical condition but then discloses a behavioral health symptom as part of the visit—for example, they come in with a headache but then also ask about an anxiety medication—they do *not* meet criteria for mandatory suicide screening. However, if there is any doubt at all about whether or not it would be helpful, it never hurts to administer the screen.

Outpatient clinicians should pay special attention to Elements of Performance (EPs) 2, 3, and 4. EP2 is the requirement that clinicians screen for suicidal ideation using an evidence-based tool (as opposed to simply just instructing clinicians to ask about suicidal ideation, which can be performed in variable ways across practices and therefore can result in variable accuracy). Examples of evidence-based screening tools suggested by TJC include the Columbia-Suicide Severity Rating Scale (C-SSRS) and the Ask Suicide Questionnaire (ASQ) Suicide Risk Screening Tool [31]. TJC also considers the PHQ-9 to be satisfactory for meeting this EP (since question #9 relates to suicidal ideation), but relying on the PHQ-9 as a suicide screen can be problematic. The PHQ-9 was designed to screen for and assess the severity of depression, of which suicidal ideation can be a symptom. While a positive response to question #9 is associated with both depression severity and long-term suicide risk, it is neither sensitive nor specific for predicting acute suicide risk and should not be interpreted as such [32, 33]. For this reason, I do not recommend using the PHQ-9 as a suicide risk screen, and any positive or negative results to question #9 should be followed up with another screening method that is more predictive of acute risk.

The C-SSRS Screener Version, summarized in Table 7.4, is a more valid tool for predicting *acute* suicide risk [34]. Anyone can be trained to use it, and it is used in a wide variety of settings both within and outside of health care systems. The screener is instructed to ask a series of three questions (1, 2 and 6) pertaining to a wish to be dead or an ambivalence about living, thoughts or fantasies about actively seeking death, and any previous suicidal behaviors, respectively. If the individual who is receiving the screen answers affirmatively to the first two questions, the screener is also instructed to ask the remaining questions 3, 4, and 5 regarding the intensity and immediacy of suicide risk. More comprehensive information about the

Table 7.4 Questions from the C-SSRS Screener Version [34]

Question	Content	Associated risk level
1	Wish to be dead	Low
2	Non-specific active suicidal thoughts	Low
3	Active suicidal ideation with any methods (not plan) without intent to act	Moderate
4	Active suicidal ideation with some intent to act, without specific plan	High
5	Active suicidal ideation with specific plan and intent	High
6	Suicidal behavior	Variable

C-SSRS as well as training materials can be found at the Columbia Lighthouse Project website, https://cssrs.columbia.edu.

The Ask Suicide-Screening Questions (ASQ) Toolkit is a similar brief screening instrument that can be found at https://www.nimh.nih.gov/research/research-conducted-at-nimh/asq-toolkit-materials.

For the purposes of this screening process—which requires "coding" recent or distant past suicidal behaviors—it is important to clarify that a suicide attempt is *any behavior taken that results in a potential for self-harm and a greater than 0% intention or expectation of dying.* Ambivalence about dying in the context of a suicide attempt is extremely common, but it is not necessarily protective [35]. At the same time, many individuals engage in self-injurious, or potentially self-injurious, behaviors without any intention to die at all, and this kind of behavior is less predictive of acute suicide risk—although even a total lack of intention or expectation to die does not guarantee survival.

For example, an individual who has ingested 100 tablets of trazodone 50 mg in an attempt to die and is rescued and resuscitated has made a suicide attempt. A different individual who has ingested five tablets of trazodone 50 mg and later says that he "wondered what would happen" has also made a suicide attempt, even though it was a much less dangerous one than in the first example. A third individual who ingested five tablets of trazodone 50 mg after researching its safety profile and determining that this dose was within the therapeutic range for depression but wanted to "scare" his partner has *not* made a suicide attempt because he had a 0% intention of dying from this—even though if he had happened to have a prolonged QTc already or was taking other QTc-prolonging medications, this might have proven more dangerous than he realized. It should also be reiterated that any information that contradicts the patient's report is fair game for consideration. If the third patient's partner subsequently produces a suicide note written by the patient and a calculation that more than five tablets of trazodone are missing from his supply, you might reasonably conclude that the third patient has also made a suicide attempt.

The genius of the C-SSRS and similar tools it is that they can be also be used to rapidly screen for and triage acute suicide risk when a concern arises either out of the screening process itself or in the course of usual clinical care. Consider the following case of a patient with a (potentially) very different risk profile from that of KG:

AT is a 72-year-old woman with COPD, coronary artery disease, hypertension, hyperlipidemia, chronic lower extremity pain, and anxiety who has grown progressively disabled over time as her symptoms have increasingly made it difficult for her to leave her home, which is on the second floor of a walk-up. She is followed closely by a care management nurse because she requires a great number of social services as well as transportation coordination for her frequent medical appointments—and frequent emergency department visits. Her nurse pages you in the middle of a clinic day to say that he just got off the phone with AT and that during their conversation, AT said, "I might as well throw myself down the stairs." You have never known her to be depressed or suicidal before. Then the nurse says, "What should we do?"

In the absence of a valid screening tool, this ambiguous statement about the stairs may need your immediate attention. After all, AT could have meant anything by that statement, and it is possible that if you delay too long in responding, you may miss an opportunity to save her life. The potential urgency of this problem might lead you to disrupt your schedule in an attempt to reach her by phone yourself (which is not the end of the world, but it comes with other tradeoffs and implications for other patients) or possibly send her—again—to the emergency department. Then again, if this statement were made flippantly, all this urgency on the part of you and your clinical team would be unnecessary.

There is an inherent problem to statements like the one that AT made, and many others that pertain to suicide: taken in isolation, and out of context, they do not provide a lot of meaningful information. The phrase, "I'm going to kill myself," can mean different things when uttered in different settings and by different people: "I'm frustrated," "I'm provoking you," "I truly want my life to be over," for example, and virtually anything else in between these extremes. Expecting health providers to jump into action when prompted by such a statement—*and get it right on a consistent basis*—is unrealistic.

In other words, you need more information in order to respond appropriately to AT's statement about throwing herself down the stairs because you do not automatically know what it means to her. The C-SSRS is a relatively fast, easy, and evidence-based method for collecting the information you need. For example:

You say to the nurse, "What was AT's score on the C-SSRS?" Fortunately, your clinic already has a protocol for using the C-SSRS in response to suicidal statements, and this nurse is well trained. He says, "She answered yes to question #1 but no to all the others. It's a low-risk screen."

With this information, suggesting that AT make a follow-up visit with you to discuss her frustrations, further assess her risk, and screen for other depressive symptoms, and then going on with the rest of your day, is likely a reasonable decision. You have already used an evidence-based tool to establish that she is in a low-risk category for acute suicidal behavior, and the complete assessment can take place on a non-emergent basis. This is very different from the alternative scenario:

You say to the nurse, "What was AT's score on the C-SSRS?" Fortunately, your clinic already has a protocol for using the C-SSRS in response to suicidal statements, and this nurse is well trained. He says, "She answered yes to questions #1, 2, 3, and 6 but no to all the others. It's a moderate risk."

This moderate risk score indicates a higher level of urgency. It does not necessarily mean that you need to send AT to the emergency department, but it means that she requires further assessment sooner than the next available follow-up appointment is likely to occur. This is a scenario in which you might consider trying to call her as soon as possible or enlisting other team members with the right expertise for assessing suicide risk acutely such as a social worker or a treating psychiatrist.

If she screens into a high acute risk category (see Table 7.4), that could suggest that she needs to be assessed right away in the emergency department. None of these are firm rules, however. The C-SSRS does not know your patients and is not designed to supplant your clinical judgment. Its usefulness instead is that it can help you collect the information that you need to screen for potential indicators of acute suicide risk quickly and systematically, and then move on to whichever next steps are most appropriate.

When further assessment is needed, EPs 3 and 4 similarly provide helpful directions. EP3 instructs clinicians to assess suicide risk by following an evidence-based process. Several tools are suggested, including the C-SSRS Risk Assessment Version (https://cssrs.columbia.edu/documents/risk-assessment-page/), which is more robust than the Screener Version, and the SAFE-T with C-SSRS (https://cssrs.columbia.edu/documents/safe-t-c-ssrs/) [36]. Both of these tools are freely available for download on the internet and provide a comprehensive checklist of factors to consider when conducting the risk assessment. TJC also allows organizations to adapt existing tools for their own individual use, provided that they satisfy the core criteria of EP3 (see Table 7.3). The purpose of these assessment tools is not to produce a triage "score" per se in the same way that the C-SSRS Screener Version does (although some versions do include numeric rating scales) but rather to prompt the clinician to conduct their risk assessments consistently and systematically for every patient.

The information obtained in the screening and assessment steps should then be used to determine and document whether the overall level of acute risk (EP4) as low, moderate, or high. The tools that are used may suggest certain types of interventions that are commonly associated with each risk level, but any mitigating steps remain up to the individual clinician's own judgment.

In essence, TJC has disseminated a template for a protocolized approach to suicide risk screening and assessment, which can help to ensure that suicide risk assessments are conducted objectively and consistently every time.

So let's return to KG. His score on the C-SSRS Screener Version places him in a high acute risk category, but if we were to track his score dynamically over time, we would find that this is his baseline. There is no indication from the screen that his short-term risk of suicide has changed. However, his risk is still high, so he requires further assessment.

A careful look at his non-modifiable risk factors include his demographic background and his family history of suicide. Modifiable risk factors include his depression and access to a firearm. The fact that he has never previously attempted suicide is protective.

You may not be able to change his mind about any of these things at a single visit, but a frank discussion about both his depression severity and his immediate access to a gun is called for. His claim that no further treatments for depression are worth pursuing should be challenged, and he may be willing to seek a second opinion from another psychiatrist even if you cannot personally list all of the new treatments that have been approved in the last 15 years. He may also be willing to collaborate on a safety plan and even allow a family member to hold onto his gun for a while as he thinks about his next steps. Or maybe he will not be willing to engage with you around any of those things and will reject your help instead. But even if he does, at least you will know that you have assessed and managed his risk using evidence-based methods. In other words, when he leaves your office, you should not have to wonder what you could have done differently.

References

1. Heron M. Deaths: leading causes for 2017. National Vital Statistics Reports 2019;68.
2. National Center for Health Statistics: Suicide and Self-Inflicted Injury. https://www.cdc.gov/nchs/fastats/suicide.htm. Accessed 7/29/21 at 9:39am.
3. World Health Organization. Suicide worldwide in 2019: global health estimates. Geneva; 2021.
4. O'Connor RC, Nock MK. The psychology of suicidal behavior. Lancet Psychiatry. 2014;1:73–85.
5. Raue PJ, Ghesquiere AR, Bruce ML. Suicide risk in primary care: identification and management in older adults. Curr Psychiatry Rep. 2014;16:466.
6. Miller IW, Camargo CA Jr, Arias SA, et al. Suicide prevention in an emergency department population: the ED-SAFE study. JAMA Psychiat. 2017;74:563–70.
7. American Psychiatric Association. Practice guideline for the assessment and treatment of patients with suicidal behaviors. 2010.
8. Florentine JB, Crane C. Suicide prevention by limiting access to methods: a review of theory and practice. Soc Sci Med. 2010:1626–32.
9. Klonsky ED, May AM, Saffer BY. Suicide, suicide attempts, and suicidal ideation. Annu Rev Clin Psychol. 2016;12:307–30.
10. Kaufman EJ, Morrison CN, Branas CC, et al. State firearm laws and interstate firearm deaths from homicide and suicide in the United States: a cross-sectional analysis of data by county. JAMA Intern Med. 2018;178:692–700.
11. Houtsma C, Butterworth SE, Anestis MD. Firearm suicide: pathways to risk and methods of prevention. Curr Opin Psychol. 2018;22:7–11.
12. Nock MK, Borges G, Bromet EJ, et al. Suicide and suicidal behavior. Epidemiol Rev. 2008;30:133–54.
13. Ribeiro JD, Franklin JC, Fox KR, et al. Self-injurious thoughts and behaviors as risk factors for future suicide ideation, attempts, and death: a meta-analysis of longitudinal studies. Psychol Med. 2016;46:225–36.
14. Franklin JC, Ribeiro JD, Fox KR, et al. Risk factors for suicidal thoughts and behaviors: a meta-analysis of 50 years of research. Psychol Bull. 2017;143:187–232.
15. McCall WV, Benca RM, Rosenquist PB, et al. Reducing suicidal ideation through insomnia treatment (REST-IT): a randomized clinical trial. Am J Psychiatr. 2019;11:957–65.

16. Stone DM, Simon TR, Fowler KA, et al. *Vital signs:* trends in state suicide rates—United States, 1999–2016 and circumstances contributing to suicide—27 states, 2015. MMWR Morb Mortal Wkly Rep. 2018;67:617–24.
17. Busch KA, Fawcett J, Jacobs DG. Clinical correlates of inpatient suicide. J Clin Psychiatry. 2003;64:14–9.
18. Madsen T, Erlangsen A, Hjorthøj C, Nordentoft M. High suicide rates during psychiatric inpatient stay and shortly after discharge. Acta Psychiatr Scand. 2020;142:355–65.
19. Lawrence RE, Perez-Cost MM, Bailey JL, et al. Coercion and the inpatient treatment alliance. Psychiatr Serv. 2019;70:1110–5.
20. Pauker SG, Kassirer JP. The threshold approach to clinical decision making. N Engl J Med. 1980;302:1109–17.
21. Glober N, Tainter CR, Brennan J, et al. Use of the D-dimer for detecting pulmonary embolism in the emergency department. J Emerg Med. 2018;54:585–92.
22. Hugli O, Righini M, Le Gal G, et al. The pulmonary embolism rule-out criteria (PERC) rule does not safely exclude pulmonary embolism. J Thromb Haemost. 2011;9:300–4.
23. DeCou CR, Comtois KA, Landes SJ. Dialectical behavior therapy is effective for the treatment of suicidal behavior: a meta-analysis. Behav Ther. 2019;50:6–72.
24. Jobes DA, Au JS, Siegelman A. Psychological approaches to suicide treatment and prevention. Curr Treat Options Psych. 2015;2:363–70.
25. D'Anci KE, Uhl S, Giradi G, Martin C. Treatments for the prevention and management of suicide: a systematic review. Ann Intern Med. 2019;171:334–42.
26. Weissman CR, Blumberger DM, Brown PE, et al. Bilateral repetitive transcranial magnetic stimulation decreases suicidal ideation in depression. J Clin Psychiatry. 2018;79:17m1111692.
27. Phillips JL, Norris S, Talbot J, et al. Single and repeated ketamine infusions for reduction of suicidal ideation in treatment-resistant depression. Neuropsychopharmacology. 2020;45:606–12.
28. Song J, Sjölander A, Joas E, et al. Suicidal behavior during lithium and valproate treatment: a within-individual 8-year prospective study of 50,000 patients with bipolar disorder. Am J Psychiatry. 2017;8:795–802.
29. Stanley B, Brown GK, Brenner LA, et al. Comparison of the safety planning intervention with follow-up vs usual care of suicidal patients treated in the emergency department. JAMA Psychiat. 2018;75:894–900.
30. Stanley B, Brown GK. Safety planning intervention: a brief intervention to mitigate suicide risk. Cogn Behav Pract. 2012;19:256–64.
31. The Joint Commission. R³ Report: National Patient Safety Goal for suicide prevention. Updated 11/20/2019. https://www.jointcommission.org/-/media/tjc/documents/standards/r3-reports/r3_18_suicide_prevention_hap_bhc_cah_11_4_19_final1.pdf, accessed 10/6/21 at 7:35pm.
32. Na PJ, Yaramala SR, Kim JA, et al. The PHQ-9 item 9 based screening for suicide risk: a validation study of the patient health questionnaire (PHQ)-9 item 9 with the Columbia Suicide Severity Rating Scale (C-SSRS). J Affect Disord. 2018;232:34–40.
33. Simon GE, Rutter CM, Peterson D, et al. Does response on the PHQ-9 depression questionnaire predict subsequent suicide attempt or suicide death? Psychiatr Serv. 2013;64(12):1195–202.
34. Posner K, Brown GK, Stanley B, et al. The Columbia-Suicide Severity Rating Scale: initial validity and internal consistency findings from three multisite studies with adolescents and adults. Am J Psychiatry. 2011;168:1266–77.
35. Macintyre VG, Mansell W, Pratt D, Tai SJ. The psychological pathway to suicide attempts: a strategy of control without awareness. Front Psychol. 2021;12:588683.
36. The Joint Commission. Suicide Prevention Resources to support Joint Commission Accredited organizations implementation of NPSG 15.01.01: EP3,4 – Validated/Evidence-Based Suicide Risk Assessment Tools. https://www.jointcommission.org/-/media/tjc/documents/resources/patient-safety-topics/suicide-prevention/pages-from-suicide_prevention_compendium_5_11_20_updated-july2020_ep3_4.pdf, accessed 10/10/21 at 10:15am.

Chapter 8
Managing Conflict

Having a depressive disorder does not make a patient difficult. However, true to our acknowledgement that depression is highly heterogeneous and multifactorial, several conditions that frequently underlie difficult patient-clinician encounters and conflict can also cause depression, and therefore clinicians who commonly treat depression should expect to sometimes need to confront situations that they find difficult or challenging.

Depression has been found to correlate with the kinds of situations that clinicians often describe as "difficult interactions" and with patients who are labeled as "difficult patients" [1–4]. Some of this association may be due to specific diagnoses in which certain kinds of events or situations are more common—for example, borderline personality disorder and frequent angry outbursts, substance use disorders and deception and denial, and somatoform disorders and demands for unnecessary medical care. However, interpersonal interactions, by definition, involve at least two people, and clinician factors can also play a role in making encounters more difficult than they need to be [2, 5].

So while it is true that some patients do not behave according to the rules that we prescribe for them, that many of these patients also have depression, and that their failing to behave "appropriately" often makes providing clinical care more difficult or even unpleasant at times, there is much that we can do to make the situation better. We also need to acknowledge that medical systems, which usually operate within a rigid structure for delivering care, can be uniquely high-risk environments for patients who have already been marginalized by other social structures. Reacting too negatively to these patients can reinforce these structural inequities and do more overall harm than good [6, 7].

It is therefore imperative that clinicians move beyond the idea of tolerating "the hateful patient" described by Groves in the seminal 1978 New England Journal of Medicine article of that name, and instead begin to understand conflict and disruption in the course of clinical practice as a confluence of many complex factors that are both personal and structural [8, 9]. Some of it may truly be the patient's fault,

D. S. Kroll, *Caring for Patients with Depression in Primary Care*, https://doi.org/10.1007/978-3-031-08495-9_8

some of it may be the clinician's fault, and all of it may be society's fault. But clinicians are usually held to a higher standard.

This does not mean that you should let your patients dictate their care or walk all over you. Setting limits is important, and this can still be done in a way that is both compassionate and effective at the same time. Consider the following case:

Ms. Wallis is a 49-year-old woman who transferred to your care about a month ago, after her previous primary care provider retired. She has a chronic history of both depression and anxiety, and her symptoms have never really improved despite "trying everything." She also has a history of alcohol use disorder, but she says that this has been in remission for the last four years.

She tells you that she feels severely depressed on a daily basis, and she is no longer working after being granted Social Security Disability benefits for her major depressive disorder and generalized anxiety disorder. Her social life is also very constricted, although she has an adult daughter who visits her about once a week.

At the time of her transfer, her medications for depression and anxiety included duloxetine 60 mg twice daily, escitalopram 20 mg daily, bupropion XL 450 mg daily, trazodone 100-200 mg daily at bedtime, clonazepam 2 mg three times daily, and gabapentin 800 mg three times daily. Her last primary care provider had been the one prescribing these medications, and she explains that she had a "bad experience" with seeing a psychiatrist and a therapist in the past. She made it clear that she expected you to take over all of these prescriptions now, and she made a comment to the effect of, "We're not going to get along well" if you did not agree to this plan.

You did not agree to this plan exactly, although there had been a lot to cover at the first visit because Ms. Wallis also has diabetes, anemia that needs to be worked up, and chronic pain, and she smokes cigarettes. You settled on a compromise, which was to educate her about the unfavorable risk/benefit ratio of taking 6 mg of clonazepam per day and to insist that tapering it (gradually) was necessary for safe care. You agreed to start by decreasing her dose to 4 mg per day (1 mg twice daily and 2 mg at bedtime) and instructed her to return in 1 month. She was less than pleased with this compromise, but after a prolonged discussion—which delayed the rest of your day by about 20 minutes—she finally agreed to leave your office. On her way out, she warned you that she did not think that she would be able to sleep on a lower dose of clonazepam and that if she wasn't sleeping, you would be hearing about it.

And you certainly have heard about it. In the last month, she has paged you first thing in the morning no fewer than eight times, insisting that you return her call immediately. Each time you have returned her call, it has involved repeating the same 15-min conversation about the inappropriateness of high-dose benzodiazepines in her care and listening to her complain about how she can't function if she doesn't sleep and about how you are making her depression worse by refusing to prescribe a treatment that has worked well enough for years. You had started to wonder whether she was right about her previous treatment regimen's stabilizing impact and had begun to doubt your own judgment about insisting on what you considered to be a safer plan. However, since she subsequently paged you at home in the evening and seemed to be slurring her words as she complained about how you were not listening to her when she was trying to tell you what she really needed, even though she continued to deny drinking, you have felt more confident with your approach.

There is a lot to unpack here. Part of what makes this case challenging is that it is easy to imagine that Ms. Wallis's next visit is going to involve a rehash of the same argument that has been driving the excessive calls and pages over the last month and that this will feel frustrating, unproductive, and highly unpleasant. Trying to set a limit with Ms. Wallis about these excessive contacts may also provoke further conflict, although it will be necessary to do so. It would be entirely reasonable for the clinician to feel a sense of dread about this upcoming appointment, and the detrimental effects of difficult patient encounters on clinician well-being and burnout should not be ignored. However, opening with an argument about why the clinician needs to be protected from Ms. Wallis's increasingly toxic behavior in order to preserve her own sanity is likely to be a losing strategy, at least with Ms. Wallis. It will also fail to address the underlying problem, which is that she is trying to strongarm her clinician into providing her with *bad care.*

A better opening strategy for breaking this problem down into manageable pieces is to **frame it from the patient's perspective**. This may seem obvious when you are withholding a treatment that is unsafe, but maintaining this framework will serve you well as you form a complete strategy. At the end of the day, Ms. Wallis's health is her problem, and the clinician is presumably in this business to help her get the best outcome she possibly can. The patient may have a narrow view about what a good health outcome looks like, and the narrowness of that perspective is likely driving what seems to be a desperate attempt to control what kind of care is provided to her. But it is almost always possible find at least some common ground (see Fig. 8.1).

Ms. Wallis has many reasonable goals, but she is distorting the importance of one aspect of her health over others—i.e., access to a supratherapeutic dose of

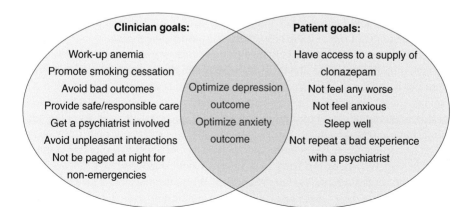

Fig. 8.1 Finding the overlap between patient and clinician goals

clonazepam [10] and all of the perceived benefits that go along with it—and prioritizing that aspect inappropriately. This is not a tradeoff that many clinicians would recommend or feel comfortable in supporting. In other words, Ms. Wallis's proposed treatment plan is targeted toward an upside-down set of priorities, and agreeing to it is not in her overall best interests, even if it is what she wants. There are many reasons for this, but a few important ones that you might emphasize include:

1. It isn't safe. Patients taking benzodiazepines at doses that are above therapeutic dosing ranges are unlikely to benefit from them and have a higher risk of adverse outcomes, which can include death [10–12].
2. It isn't effective. Benzodiazepines are not associated with better long-term outcomes in anxiety disorders and are not recommended for long-term use [13, 14]. They also are not effective for depression and may instead lead to worse outcomes [15].
3. It isn't effective *for her*. This is important! She has not achieved a good outcome for either her depression or her anxiety, which have become chronic and associated with low social and occupational functioning levels. The outcome she is currently getting is not satisfactory and should not be accepted as an endpoint of treatment.

The third point, of course, is the one with the most immediate impact on Ms. Wallis, and it may resonate with her better than the first two, which may be perceived as too abstract or defensive. It is an argument that directly applies to her condition, and it is therefore a more powerful one. She is not doing well with the status quo, and therefore the clinician in the vignette is not willing to perpetuate it.

The high-dose benzodiazepine is not the only problem, however. Ms. Wallis is also asking the clinician to maintain an overall treatment regimen that is complicated, likely suboptimal, and high-risk on multiple fronts, and at the same time, she is choosing the wrong setting for her care. While of course, depression, anxiety, and alcohol use disorder can all be managed safely and effectively in primary care, primary care is not the best setting for Ms. Wallis's treatment plan. Why? Because the rationale and long-term plan for each component of her current treatment is not clear.

Notice here that I did not say that primary care is not the best setting for Ms. Wallis. I said that it was not the best setting for her *treatment plan*.

Part of the goal of this book is to help primary care providers become more comfortable to both *implement* and *understand* appropriate treatment plans for depression. For a patient with recurrent major depressive disorder to take bupropion XL 300 mg once daily as part of a long-term plan *makes sense*. It is consistent with both treatment guidelines and conventional practices. Conversely, it is unlikely that any clinician would automatically know how Ms. Wallis's treatment plan came about based on her diagnoses. Why is she taking an SSRI and SNRI together and at maximum doses? Why does she need high doses of both trazodone and clonazepam? What is the target symptom for her gabapentin? Why can't she work with a therapist?

There is a possibility that a reasonable rationale for this treatment plan exists, but that rationale is not obvious. The clinician should acknowledge their own lack of understanding because it is *a fact that cannot be argued with*.

Medical facts are often easy to challenge. Medical literature does not provide a consistent, coherent message about every subject, and medical scholars are—and should be—constantly challenging each other and conventional wisdom. No wonder, then, that in this era in which many patients come into their visits armed with their own independent research, they are not always easy to convince of something that they do not already believe [9]. Some of them may even legitimately have more information memorized than you do about some topics.

Making an argument based on scientific evidence may convince some patients but may engender debate in others. While this is healthy and maybe even desirable in some circumstances, this approach has been counterproductive with Ms. Wallis so far. For every reason you list in support of your concerns about her treatment plan being unsafe, she can probably find a reason—or maybe even an article—that says otherwise.

But this is not a logic contest. The root of the issue is that the clinician does not feel comfortable with the plan and is more attuned to the obvious risks than to the not-so-clear benefits. And the clinician (hopefully) has a license to protect. At first glance, this seems to place the clinician in the awkward position of having to decide between acceding to a treatment plan that she does not agree with and perpetuating the conflict with the patient—and all of the practical challenges that go along with it.

But it is also a fixable problem—and one that, in fact, the clinician and the patient share together. The patient is asking for a treatment plan that the clinician is not comfortable offering. Using the mutual problem as a starting point—rather than the proposed "solutions" that are in conflict—can open up more opportunities for a reasonable compromise.

Solutions that could be considered for this problem include:

1. The clinician could change her comfort level with all or some aspects of the treatment plan. I would not recommend this as a first-choice solution in this particular case, but there are some situations in which this option could be desirable. For example, if a clinician is not comfortable with a particular (reasonable) treatment modality because of a fixable knowledge gap (e.g., he or she has never prescribed vortioxetine, and usually doesn't, but inherits a patient who is benefiting from it), the comfort level could be an appropriate target for problem-solving.
2. The patient could change her priorities. Good luck with this! But sometimes providing education and advice to patients actually does work.
3. The patient could accept a referral to a psychiatrist. This is more than simply passing the buck to another clinician. It is making a referral to a specialist in a situation where a specialist is likely to have a higher degree of expertise for managing a particular set of problems.

Anyone who has read the 1983 classic book on negotiating, *Getting to Yes*, may recognize this strategy as analogous to what its authors called "principled negotiation" [16]. Principled negotiation refers to the idea that conflict should be approached from the standpoint of trying to fix a problem or set of problems rather than trying to push for a particular solution. It is common for people to assume that a "victory" in negotiating means leaving the table with everything they asked for when they came to it (i.e., positional negotiation), and sometimes this is possible to do, particularly when one party has significantly more power or motivation than the other. However, tying the idea of success to one particular outcome in conflict resolution is inherently inflexible and usually implies that there should be both a winner and a loser. It is also more difficult to "win" in this framework when neither party has any real control over what the other does. All too often, negotiations break down, or one or both of the parties eventually gets worn down by the other and gives in.

Focusing on the problem rather than a particular solution from the outset allows more opportunity for finding a creative compromise that satisfies all parties. Here, solution #3 seems like a highly reasonable one. Ms. Wallis might even accept it outright, or she might not. The clinician cannot force her to. However, no matter what she chooses to do, the framework for a treatment plan has been set: the specific medication regimen she is asking for requires a psychiatrist's involvement.

The reverse of this is also true: by insisting that a certain treatment plan requires a specialist, the clinician is also acknowledging that assuming responsibility for the psychiatric treatment plan in primary care would necessitate a different treatment plan. It is replacing a "no" answer with a "yes, and." Instead of saying, "I won't prescribe your psychiatric medications," the clinician is saying, "If I were to prescribe your psychiatric medications, this is what it would look like." Her medication regimen would not involve every medication that she is asking for but would instead be simpler and more transparently evidence-based.

Let's assume for a moment that Ms. Wallis is still refusing to accept a psychiatry referral, even after the clinician has made a compelling case for it. Maybe she even has a good reason, or maybe there are simply no psychiatrists who are willing to take her case. Whether or not it is her "fault" is irrelevant. Providing a safer, more evidence-based treatment plan is not a punishment. So how does one actually do this?

First, it might be helpful to systematically break down each element of the medication regimen into what you already know to be major risks, potential treatment targets in general, and likely treatment targets as they apply specifically to Ms. Wallis. As you do this, acknowledge where there may be gaps in your knowledge. Then, look for evidence that each medication has been helpful or not. Table 8.1 illustrates this process.

Systematically considering each part of this regimen creates a pretty bleak picture for Ms. Wallis's overall treatment plan. She is taking a lot of different medications, and the benefits from this treatment have been limited so far. She may even benefit from a total treatment plan overhaul. But that is not her most immediate need. The first order of business is to minimize the amount of risk associated with her current plan while avoiding any steps that are likely to completely destabilize her.

Her clonazepam dose should be reduced to a therapeutic range (cutoffs for this are not universally agreed upon, but a maximum of 2 mg/day is a reasonable threshold) [12], although it may not be safe to discontinue it outright. She should be offered a gradual taper, which could take several months or even longer, depending

Table 8.1 Systematically breaking down a complex treatment regimen

Medication	Possible indications	Likely indications in Ms. Wallis	Major concerns	Evidence it is working
Escitalopram	Depression, anxiety	Depression, anxiety	Interaction with duloxetine and trazodone	No clear benefit
Duloxetine	Depression, anxiety, chronic pain	Depression, anxiety, chronic pain	Interaction with escitalopram and trazodone	No clear benefit
Bupropion	Depression, smoking	Depression, maybe smoking?		No clear benefit
Trazodone	Sleep, depression	Sleep	Interaction with escitalopram and duloxetine	Subjectively says it helps with sleep
Clonazepam	Anxiety, sleep, restless legs syndrome	Sleep, anxiety	Supratherapeutic dose, long-term use, alcohol use disorder	Subjectively says it helps with sleep and appetite
Gabapentin	Neuropathic pain, anxiety	Unclear	Unclear indication, risk of abuse	No clear indication or benefit

on the acuity of her risk and how well she tolerates it [17]. Decreasing the dose to 4 mg/day as a starting point is likely a good balance between the many competing priorities.

Gabapentin should be discontinued unless a clear indication for it can be identified. Although it is sometimes used off-label for anxiety disorders, it is not considered to be first-line treatment for anxiety, and it is not clear why this would be needed on top of her existing regimen [18]. There is also some abuse potential associated with gabapentin, and it should not be assumed that this risk is not relevant to Ms. Wallis [19]. If becomes clear from this discussion that gabapentin is intended to treat Ms. Wallis's pain, and not her anxiety, the clinician can then determine whether it makes sense to also think about her treatment plan for pain systematically and consider additional referrals if needed.

Neither duloxetine nor escitalopram is problematic on its own, but these should not be combined at maximum therapeutic doses along with trazodone due to this combination being a relatively high risk one for serotonin toxicity. She should therefore choose one or the other, keeping in mind also that there could be cumulative effects from escitalopram and trazodone on prolonging the QTc interval [20]. If neither has been effective for depression or anxiety, both could be tapered.

Whether there has been any further benefit from the addition of bupropion to the SSRI or SNRI is probably debatable, but a combination of an SSRI or SNRI with bupropion is at least evidence-based. If it was intended for depression (as opposed to smoking cessation), maintaining it as part of a holding pattern until Ms. Wallis connects with psychiatry is reasonable. If it was intended to treat smoking cessation, it has not been effective in doing so; unless Ms. Wallis has noticed some collateral benefit for depression in the process, it should be discontinued.

This example is intended to illustrate a process rather than a specific outcome. For real patients, there may be other factors that shift the risk/benefit ratios of specific decisions, and there may also be other priorities that compete with any problems in the psychiatric treatment plan and end up becoming more pressing, particularly at the initial visit. But the take-home point is that clinicians should not allow themselves to be strongarmed into providing care that they are not comfortable with and do not understand when reasonable alternatives and/or compromises can be identified.

Anyway, we're not done. The clinician in this case still needs to address the excessive phone calls, which could get worse as increasing limits are set on the treatment plan. But the approach to this problem is not too different from how the first conflict about medications was addressed. Although a great argument could be made about how Ms. Wallis's behavior is negatively impacting the clinician and probably the rest of the clinic staff, that argument is likely to fall flat. Not that it isn't important—staff burnout can have serious consequences for patient care (see Table 8.2). Nonetheless, the argument that is most likely to resonate with Ms. Wallis is the one that persuades her that this behavior is *not in her own best interests.*

Excessively calling and paging clinicians about non-emergent issues is not only distracting and bothersome—it is *ineffective.* Most clinical paging systems are set up to facilitate the communication of urgent information, and this is how they perform best. Using the paging system for other purposes weakens that system and can lead to alarm fatigue. At the same time, it bypasses the team-based care structure that modern clinical systems depend on in order to deliver consistent, safe, and reliable care.

When a patient bypasses usual protocols in order to get a particular clinician's attention more quickly and directly, this opens up more room for error. Alarm fatigue on its own can lead to more mistakes, and when a channel for urgent communications is diluted by non-urgent annoyances, this can make it more difficult to triage these alarms appropriately [29]. Keep in mind that clinicians typically are not just sitting in a room and waiting for the calls to come in. Deciding when and if to respond to a page usually requires making a tradeoff between different competing priorities. If you have another pressing situation (or another patient) in front of you, and a page comes in that has a > 90% chance of being non-urgent based on historical precedent, it would be rational to triage your attention away from that "alarm" and toward the other situation instead. Meanwhile, there is usually very little systemic support to ensure that clinicians remember later to return to all the pages that they did not respond to when they first came in.

Table 8.2 Clinician-facing and patient-facing consequences of burnout among clinicians [21–28]	Patient-centered	Clinician-centered
	More clinical errors	Lower job satisfaction
	Lower quality of care	Compassion fatigue
	Decreased professionalism	Depression
	Decreased compassion	Substance abuse
		Job turnover

On the other hand, if a patient calls a clinic with a question or concern, clinics usually have team-based protocols to ensure that those communications are handled in a systematic way to reduce the chance of their being forgotten or lost in the shuffle. The main clinical provider or team leader may not always respond to each patient directly, but the tradeoff is that patients get the care they need more reliably. It also acknowledges that the clinical provider or team leader is not always going to be the most effective individual to respond to every kind of request.

For example, if a patient calls a clinician directly in order to schedule an appointment, and that clinician does not have immediate access to the schedule, the clinician will need to go through several extra steps, including some that involve waiting for other staff members to respond, in order to complete that request. It is a slower process, and in the meantime, another patient might call the scheduling team in the correct way and take the spot that the clinician promised the first patient. Then everyone has to start over.

Patients who challenge the team-based care structure of modern clinical settings therefore need to understand that the team exists not just to insulate clinicians from their patients but instead to ensure that patients get what they need in the timeliest and most accurate manner possible. A side effect is that clinician time is also freed up in order to provide direct care to a higher volume of patients and ultimately expand health care access to a broader population.

The conversation with Ms. Wallis, then, might go something like this:

After they finished discussing Ms. Wallis's medical treatment plan—which was not an easy conversation, but it was a productive one—you add, "We also need to talk about the extra phone calls and pages I've been getting from you in the last few weeks. That's not the right way to communicate with me."

Ms. Wallis interrupts, "I told you that I need to sleep. Sleep is very important to me."

You've got this. You calmly respond, "I understand that, but calling me to let me know about every bad night's sleep you get is not helping things. A phone call like that is not the right setting for making a change in your treatment plan, and it's also creating a pattern where I already don't know how to triage your calls anymore. When I get a message that something is urgent, that usually means I need to drop whatever I'm doing and take care of that message immediately, but if you're telling me that everything is urgent, then I don't know what it means when you say that. Eventually, I'm going to miss something important. Plus, I'm not always available to call you back, and if you're waiting for me specifically every time, you may be waiting longer than you need to, especially if it really is important or could be handled better by another person. We have a whole team in place to ensure that you don't get stuck waiting and that important things don't get missed. I need to insist that you take advantage of that team and go through the usual channels when you have a clinical question."

"But you're my doctor, and I expect and need you to be available when I call," Ms. Wallis says.

"My priority is providing you with good medical care, and good medical care means that we follow procedures and work in teams.

Hopefully, this case effectively illustrates how clinicians can approach conflicts from the patient's perspective and feel comfortable that setting limits is not just about self-care. It is an essential part of providing high quality care to patients, even if they are asking you to provide something different.

References

1. Kroenke K. Patients presenting with somatic complaints: epidemiology, psychiatric co-morbidity and management. Int J Methods Psychiatr Res. 2003;12:34–43.
2. Hinchey SA, Jackson JL. A cohort study assessing difficult patient encounters in a walk-in primary care clinic, predictors and outcomes. J Gen Intern Med. 2011;26:588–94.
3. Jackson JL, Kroenke K. Difficult patient encounters in the ambulatory clinic: clinical predictors and outcomes. Arch Intern Med. 1999;159:1069–75.
4. Hahn SR, Kroenke K, Spitzer RL, et al. The difficult patient: prevalence, psychopathology, and functional impairment. J Gen Intern Med. 1996;11:1–8.
5. Krebs EE, Garrett JM, Konrad TR. The difficult doctor? Characteristics of physicians who report frustration with patients: an analysis of survey data. BMC Health Serv Res. 2006;6:128.
6. Legemaate J. Involuntary discharge of voluntary psychiatric patients. Med Law. 1991;10:363–8.
7. McNeil R, Small W, Wood E, Kerr T. Hospitals as a 'risk environment': an ethno-epidemiologic study of voluntary and involuntary discharge from hospitals against medical advice among people who inject drugs. Soc Sci Med. 2014;105:59–66.
8. Groves JE. Taking care of the hateful patient. NEJM. 1978;298:883–7.
9. Strous RD, Ulman A, Kotler M. The hateful patient revisited: relevance for 21st century medicine. Eur J Intern Med. 2006;17:387–93.
10. Cushman P, Benzer D. Benzodiazepines and drug abuse: clinical observations in chemically dependent persons before and during abstinence. Drug Alcohol Depend. 1980;6:365–71.
11. Kripke DF, Langer RD, Kline LE. Hypnotics' association with mortality and cancer: a matched cohort study. BMJ Open. 2012;2:e000850.
12. Kroll DS, Nieva HR, Barsky AJ, Linder JA. Benzodiazepines are prescribed more frequently to patients already at risk for benzodiazepine-related adverse events in primary care. J Gen Intern Med. 2016;31:1027–34.
13. Moore N, Pariente A, Bégaud B. Why are benzodiazepines not yet controlled substances? JAMA Psychiat. 2015;72:110–1.
14. Olfson M, King M, Scheonbaum M. Benzodiazepine use in the United States. JAMA Psychiat. 2015;72:136–42.
15. Lim B, Sproul BA, Zahra Z, et al. Understanding the effects of chronic benzodiazepine use in depression: a focus on neuropharmacology. Int Clin Psychopharmacol. 2020;35:243–53.
16. Fisher R, Ury W. Getting to yes. Penguin Books; 1983.
17. Lader M. Benzodiazepine harm: how can it be reduced? Br J Clin Pharmacol. 2014;77:295–301.
18. Garakini A, Murrough JW, Freire RC, et al. Pharmacotherapy of anxiety disorders: current emerging treatment options. Front Psych. 2020;11:595584.
19. Smith RV, Havens JR, Walsh SL. Gabapentin misuse, abuse and diversion: a systematic review. Addiction. 2016;111:1160–74.
20. Beach SR, Kostis WJ, Celano CM, et al. Meta-analysis of selective serotonin reuptake inhibitor-associated QTc prolongation. J Clin Psychiatry. 2014;75:e441–9.
21. Al Hariri M, Hamade B, Bizri M, et al. Psychological impact of COVID-19 on emergency department healthcare workers in a tertiary care center during a national economic crisis. Am J Emerg Med. 2022;51:342–7.
22. Vose JM. Addressing stress and burnout in hematology/oncology physicians. Oncology. 2021:520.

23. Alabi RO, Hietanen P, Elmusrati M, et al. Mitigating burnout in an oncological unit: a scoping review. Front Public Health. 2021;9:677915.

24. Owoc J, Manczak M, Jablonska M, et al. Association between physician burnout and self-reported errors: meta-analysis. J Patient Saf. 2022;18:e180–8

25. Berger RS, White RJ, Faith MA, Stapleton S. Compassion fatigue in pediatric hematology, oncology, and bone marrow transplant healthcare providers: an integrative review. Palliat Support Care. 2021;

26. Brenner MJ, Hickson GB, Boothman RC, et al. Honesty and transparency, indispensable to the clinical mission—part III. How leaders can prevent burnout, foster wellness and recovery, and instill resilience. Otolaryngol Clin N Am. 2022;55:83–103.

27. Kratzke IM, Woods LC, Adapa K, et al. The sociotechnical factors associated with burnout in residents in surgical specialties: a qualitative systematic review. J Surg Educ. 2021;

28. Nituica C, Bota OA, Blebea J, et al. Factors influencing resilience and burnout among resident physicians—a national survey. BMC Med Educ. 2021;21:514.

29. Ruskin KJ, Hueske-Kraus D. Alarm fatigue: impacts on patient safety. Curr Opin Anaesthesiol. 2015;28:685–90.

Chapter 9
Disability and the Legal System

Depression is the leading cause of disability in the world [1]. Even in cases that involve primarily physical injuries, the added presence of depression is strongly associated with more severe impairment [2]. This relationship appears to be bidirectional and complex. Individuals who have developed significant physical symptoms or lost function as a result of physical injuries are likely to describe feeling depressed as a result, while pre-existing depression is a known risk factor for work injuries and disability [3]. Because many depressive disorders are chronic, individuals who have difficulty working as a result of their depressive symptoms may also require recurrent leaves of absence throughout their careers [4].

Primary care providers are—and should be—among the first people that most individuals who perceive themselves as having become disabled will turn to for help, and it is extremely likely that some patients will ask you to support claims that they can no longer work because of a depressive disorder that may or may not have occurred as a result of a work injury. Ultimately, it is not up to you to decide whether or not a patient actually returns to work or whether their disability claims lead to any benefits or compensation—unless, perhaps, you moonlight as a judge. But your opinion matters. What you advise your patients, and how you document that advice, can shape the way your patients—and any other individuals and organizations who may have a stake in this process—approach their health needs for years to come.

As your clinical care of a patient begins to intersect with a legal agenda, you may be asked to say, do, or write things in pursuit of a goal that may or may not fully align with yours (i.e., to provide the best possible health care). This can put you in a difficult position. When a patient says to you, for example, "My lawyer says I need neuropsychological testing," that does not mean that the lawyer has completed a clinical assessment and then recommended the most appropriate evidence-based workup. For you to then immediately refer the patient for testing, and in so doing indicate to his insurance company that this is clinically indicated and should be paid for, would be inappropriate. Instead, you have to rely on your own expertise (or that

D. S. Kroll, *Caring for Patients with Depression in Primary Care*, https://doi.org/10.1007/978-3-031-08495-9_9

of other clinical team members whom you trust) and do what you believe to be clinically correct.

Of course, not all disability assessments are going to be minefields. More often than not, the patient's medical and legal agendas will share at least some common goals, and it is hard to imagine many cases in which a patient says to you, "My lawyer says I should see a therapist," and you won't be able to think of any valid clinical reasons to agree with this. But there are some tricks to navigating these situations correctly. We'll use a case to illustrate them:

Gerri, a 60-year-old woman whom you have treated for hypertension for the last six years, presents to your office following a panic attack that occurred at work. She explains that she has been having a very hard time in her job as a teacher in the last two years as a result of a new principal in her school, and she has been feeling very depressed. She has taught sixth-grade English for almost twenty years, but in the last two years her principal's actions have caused her to feel undermined in her job, unsupported in the classroom, and at times unsafe. At the same time, the students in her classroom are becoming more difficult to teach every year due to their increasing oppositional behavior. In the last two months, she has cried every night after getting home from school, and she finally "just couldn't take it anymore" when an eleven-year-old student in her classroom used an insulting term about her, which caused her to have a panic attack. She was evaluated in the emergency department afterward, and she is not planning to return to her job again. She needs you to write a letter explaining that she is depressed and permanently disabled as a result of this and other incidents that have occurred in the course of her work.

In this case example, the story that Gerri relates to you in her visit is only one part of a much larger narrative. You might (or might not) find her to be very trustworthy and candid, but it is rare that any individual patient can explain a series of events such as this one in a way that is both concise and totally comprehensive, even if their intentions are honest. It is also natural for human beings to embellish the extent of their symptoms or losses in the context of explaining a potential work injury to a healthcare provider, even if they are not doing this on purpose [5]. As far as you know in this moment, a number of different explanations for Gerri's presentation might be plausible:

Scenario 1: Gerri was just trying to go about her job and essentially mind her own business when a new principal, who may have been either inept or malicious, came on board and either changed the system in a way that made Gerri's life miserable for two years or failed to adapt the system to new pressures, such as an increasing volume of students with behavioral problems.

This, it seems, is how Gerri perceives her situation, and it is most likely how a hypothetical plaintiff's attorney that she may or may not have hired, or eventually will hire, hopes that you will, too.

Scenario 2: Gerri grew tired of working as a teacher and decided to cash out by filing a frivolous lawsuit. She thinks that you are a pushover who will believe whatever she tells you, and she is counting on your unwavering support as she continues to make increasingly outlandish claims in the coming years as her case unfolds.

Malingering is common among patients who are seeking compensation for a disability claim, with some estimates suggesting that the majority of patients in this position will engage in some form of willful deception as a part of this process [5]. However, let's assume that you fundamentally do not believe this is the case for Gerri. You might be wrong—any of us can be taken advantage of—but it is not a bad thing to trust that our patients are acting in good faith most of the time.

The real truth, anyway, is usually somewhere in between these two scenarios. Patients can exaggerate or misrepresent facts related to a disability claim without deliberately trying to deceive anyone, and they may not understand critical elements of their own cases that a thorough clinical examination would uncover. For example, Gerri's work performance could have declined in recent years as a result of subtle cognitive impairments that she is not yet aware of, and she is mistakenly blaming other people for her new difficulties. Alternatively, she might have a personality disorder that has been associated with interpersonal difficulties throughout her life, and a deeper exploration would show that none of these complaints are new or unique to this current principal. Or perhaps she is more or less naturally prone to major depressive disorder, and her recent work stressors genuinely contributed either a lot or a little to her current major depressive episode.

Or maybe none of these explanations is the right one. The important point is that, from your vantage point, you cannot possibly see the whole story. *It is not your job* to see the whole story. You are a health care provider, not a detective. Your job is to provide the highest quality health care possible. In practical terms, this means that what you say to the patient and document in the record should reflect your own clinical assessment to the best of your ability, and it is OK if there are gaps in your knowledge that limit what you can and cannot say with medical certainty.

Allow these two, fairly intuitive, rules to guide you:

1. Tell the truth.
2. State as facts only what you know to be facts.

The first point should be obvious, but the second requires a little more thoughtfulness. If we just established that you do not have all of the information you need to render an opinion about this case, what is there left to document?

In fact, there is a lot that you *do* know. Even if you know very little about the true nature of your patient's work situation, you know how to perform an examination. You also know more than she does about depressive disorders and what causes them. You know at least something about your patient's medical history, family history, social circumstances, and lifestyle habits that may or may not be immediately relevant to your assessment. You know what treatments are available and appropriate for whatever condition your patient has, and you may be able to give her a fairly accurate prognosis.

Depression can cause or contribute to disability through a number of mechanisms. A severe loss of interest in one's own future, or significant apathy, can result in patients' failing to get to work at all, or in some cases failing to get out of bed, and employers will perceive this as absenteeism [6]. Impaired motivation, energy, and concentration or a significant loss of sleep can also negatively affect productivity or work quality, a phenomenon commonly referred to as "presentee-ism" [6]. Employers or supervisors may interpret these changes in work performance as a signal that the patient is a bad employee, and the patient may thus miss opportunities for advancement or even lose his or her job after receiving negative performance reviews. The usual value of taking a disability leave lies in temporarily removing the patient with severe depression from a situation in which they may perform noticeably poorly in their work and simultaneously give them the space in which to pursue evidence-based treatment and stabilize their symptoms. To say that a patient has become permanently disabled as a result of their depression means that there is no reasonable expectation that they will ever recover. In other words, the depression has become both chronic and hopelessly treatment refractory.

In this case, Gerri has asked you to write a letter, and this is a reasonable request. However, she is not a health care provider. She has framed this request from the perspective of someone who does not yet understand that a disability assessment involves more than simply accepting her statement at face value, that emotional distress does not always equal injury or disability, or that depression is often treatable. She also may not realize that you do not have the power to make a final determination regarding any benefits or compensation she will receive in the future. What she says to you requires clinical interpretation. If you agree to write this letter, it should convey that you have listened to her story, examined her, and applied a diagnosis that is reasonable and appropriate based on your objective clinical assessment.

It might look like this:

To Whom it May Concern,

I examined Ms. Gerri Jones on March 9, 2021. She reported to me that she has been feeling increasingly depressed over the last two years. She associates feeling depressed with stress she has been experiencing at work. My examination reveals her to be visibly distressed and tearful at times. I have diagnosed her with an adjustment disorder [or major depressive disorder, or bipolar disorder, etc.]*, and I have advised that she take the next four weeks off from work in order to pursue treatment.*

Notice that this letter does not describe any events that you did not personally witness, and it does not offer an opinion as to whether any work events or work stress caused her to develop an adjustment disorder. It makes it clear what Gerri told you and what you personally found on examining her. It contains only what you know to be facts—the truth, the whole truth, and nothing but the truth as far as you know. The recommendation that Gerri take several weeks off from work is somewhat arbitrary, but it reflects an expectation that the symptoms of an adjustment disorder should resolve spontaneously with time and with removal of the stressor. If you had diagnosed major depressive disorder and begun an SSRI, you might have recommended 6 or 8 weeks off from work instead, in order to allow for a full therapeutic response to treatment.

If you can say with certainty that a particular injury was, in fact, the most likely cause of the condition you have diagnosed, it is fine to say so. Some situations are more clear-cut than others, although this is more likely to be the case with physical injuries as opposed to psychiatric ones. Because most depression is multifactorial, there will usually be at least some ambiguity around causation at this early stage in the investigation.

If Gerri's claim does ultimately lead to a contest of some kind—a lawsuit against her employer or a claim against her insurance company, for example—she may be asked to meet with one or more independent medical examiners. The independent medical examiner—typically a psychiatrist in the case of a depression-related claim—evaluates the patient in a non-clinical setting for the purpose of providing an impartial assessment. Presumably, this examiner will also have access to your records as well as other materials that you may not have had the opportunity to review (including, often, the observations of private investigators who have been hired to do surveillance [5]) and will be able to render an opinion about the diagnosis and its cause based on an arguably more thorough investigation than most clinical providers are able to undertake in their practices.

However, whether or not the independent medical examiners have more information than you do that might be pertinent to attributing causation—or whether or not you agree with their assessments—they do not have a clinical role in your patients' care and have not been hired to help them get the best health outcomes. It is remarkably easy to lose sight of the fact that your goal is to help your patients to get the best health outcome possible after they—and sometimes you and your team by extension—have been sucked into the medico-legal machine. A plaintiff's attorney, for example, might have genuinely good intentions for advancing your patient's interests, but the focus of her job is not to get the best health outcomes for her client. It is to get justice. Whatever a lawyer asks you to do will likely be in pursuit of this goal, which often means some kind of compensation or benefits. Although these goals can overlap with health goals, a successful lawsuit should not be equated with successful health care.

In other words, *permanent total disability is not a good health outcome!*

This may be intuitive, but it is so easy to forget in real time. After years of visiting clinicians, lawyers, independent examiners, and courtrooms—all of which can turn into a full-time job in and of itself—some patients will receive a ruling in favor of their disability claim and be granted access to benefits and financial resources that may or may not be sufficient to compensate them for what they have lost. Others will not. The ruling may be right or wrong, or neither. But some patients have been so laser-focused on doing the work required by their lawsuit that they have allowed their treatment to fall by the wayside. The outcome of the lawsuit does not reflect the quality of care you have provided, and permanent disability—while unavoidable in some cases—should never, ever be your goal.

Instead, your first goal should be to ensure that your patients receive the best treatment possible despite the many distractions that may come up in the course of pursuing their claims. It is deceptively easy for an evidence-based treatment plan to slip away amid the overwhelming volume of social and legal obligations that disability claimants are facing. Whether or not this happens is not always under your control. The many scenarios in which patients reject or fail to follow through with treatment recommendations that exist in the course of regular clinical care apply here, too. However, the same effort that you would exert to engage a patient in

Imagine that you diagnosed a patient with major depressive disorder and prescribed an SSRI while also making a referral to psychotherapy. A year later, that patient returns to you and explains, "I never took the medication because a family member said I shouldn't, and the therapist you referred me to never called me back." Under ordinary circumstances, you would want to use this opportunity to re-evaluate the patient and try to re-engage him or her in first-line treatment for depression. But if then the patient adds, "I'm here because I need a letter stating that I'm still depressed and can't work," that can easily distract you from providing the clinical care that seemed so clearly appropriate in the previous sentence. If the patient is not asking for clinical care, you may need to be the one who speaks up about it.

Fig. 9.1 Getting distracted by the medicolegal machine

evidence-based treatment can be just as helpful in this context as it would in any other. In other words, actions that support the legal case should not take the place of providing clinical care (Fig. 9.1).

Regardless of whether or not their lawsuits are ultimately successful, individuals who are unable to work as a result of severe depression do not have a good quality of life. Not only must they bear the symptoms of severe depression (potentially for the rest of their working lives, or longer), but also are also more likely to live in poverty and to remain at an economic disadvantage even if they return to work later in their lives [7]. Younger adults who fall out of the work force temporarily, for example, lose potentially irreplaceable opportunities to lay the foundations of a successful career, and middle-aged or older adults who are disabled are unable to reap the benefits of what are likely to be their peak earning years [7, 8]. At the same time, individuals who are perceived—and perceive themselves—as disabled commonly regress to a state invalidism that makes it psychologically more difficult for them to lead productive lives even after their original injuries (whether exaggerated or not) have healed [5].

This best-case scenario of healing a patient's depression and empowering them to return to work is not always possible. Although in general, successfully returning to work is indicative of better health outcomes, this does not apply if the work environment is truly hostile or toxic. Individuals who are being bullied, harassed, or abused should not be encouraged to return to a setting in which this is likely to recur. Even if most of us would like to believe that most workplaces have safeguards in place to prevent or curtail abusive behavior, in practice we cannot always count on such safeguards being effective. In these cases, successful treatment might look different. It might mean that the patient leaves her current job but gets a new job somewhere else, or it might mean that she finds something else to do with her time that is equally meaningful. This is a part of the outcome that you cannot control, but if you are giving your patients the right kind of treatment and space to heal, they can make their own decisions about what kind of form that healing takes.

As you think about formulating the best treatment plan, consider the following pearls:

– Make sure that that you have not skipped first-line treatment (usually an antidepressant medication, psychotherapy, or both).
– If first-line treatments have not been successful, enlist the help of a specialist (if possible) before declaring the patient's condition to be treatment-refractory or permanent. Of course, you know this! But patients may declare themselves to be treatment-refractory even if they have not truly met the diagnostic criteria for treatment resistant depression, and it can be hard to keep track of this on your own, especially if the patient is visiting you only intermittently over a period of years.
– Insomnia is an especially common theme in disability cases but is often readily treatable [9]. Ask about sleep habits and consider that addressing insomnia directly could be high yield.
– Any patients who have been unemployed for prolonged periods may benefit from a gradual return to work plan rather than returning to full duty right away. Consider referring them to a vocational rehabilitation program, especially if they do not feel quite ready for a regular job [10].
– If no usual treatments are effective, reconsider the likelihood that the patient may be exaggerating symptoms. Although treatment resistant depression can occur, in the setting of a disability claim this should be considered a red flag indicating that you do not have all the information that you need. It is also important to recognize that both litigation and unemployment are highly stressful conditions that may have an ongoing impact on mood and could also explain the persistence of an adjustment disorder beyond the point at which you would have expected it to resolve.

Emotional Support Animals

The certification of patient's pet as an emotional support animal (ESA) is a special kind of disability assessment that you are also likely to be approached about.

Being asked to write a letter in support of an ESA poses a dilemma. On the one hand, this is an easy way to make some patients' lives easier. When one is being forced by his or her landlord to choose between losing his or her housing and giving up a pet, it is natural to want to find another solution, and perhaps the most expedient way to accomplish this is to ask a clinician for what is, practically speaking, a letter of protection. In the United States, the Fair Housing Act requires landlords to allow tenants to keep animals who have been certified as ESAs in their homes, and all the tenant needs to do in order to access this right is produce a letter, signed by any health care provider, to this effect [11, 12]. The other protection that is provided to ESAs (by the Air Carrier Access Act) is free passage in the cabin of an airplane, assuming, of course, that they are accompanied by their human companions [11]. That is all. ESAs are not service animals and do not have special freedoms to enter any other public spaces, no matter how much their owners might insist otherwise [12]. ESAs are also not given any special protections by the Americans with Disabilities Act [11].

At the same time, certifying an ESA is more complicated—both clinically and legally—than many clinicians realize. In addition to the fact that no clinician is likely to understand the full spectrum of consequences that might result from writing this letter—and in fact, scientific evidence to support the use of ESAs in depression or other emotional disorders is lacking [11]—this letter also constitutes a determination of disability. A letter certifying that your patient requires an ESA is, technically, a letter certifying that your patient has a psychiatric disability and that having the ESA is necessary to minimize the impact of that disability on their functioning or health [11].

There is, naturally, a great deal of fraud in this area. Many humans dress up their pets in vests and ID tags that have no legally recognized role in identifying them as either service or emotional support animals, and this can lead to a great deal of confusion among the general public around who is entitled to bring animals into public spaces, what their functions are supposed to be, and what kind of training standards they have met in order to qualify for those freedoms [12]. Meanwhile, thanks in part to this confusion and in part to relatively weak regulations on the certification process, it is easy enough for many people to obtain the letters they want online from clinicians whom they have never met.

Some groups, including the American Psychological Association, have begun to openly discourage treating clinicians from certifying ESAs on the grounds that most of them are not qualified to perform this assessment properly. The potential for unintended negative consequences is also high, and it is difficult to weigh this favorably against the fact that certifying an ESA is not considered an evidence-based treatment for any mental health disorder [12].

Potential unintended consequences of certifying an ESA can include both legal and clinical outcomes. Consider the following possibilities [11, 12]:

– Animals may become unduly stressed in unfamiliar environments (such as an airport or a plane) and then misbehave in any variety of ways.
– The rights of the ESA may conflict with the rights of other humans (or even other animals) who have not had an opportunity to plead their case to you.
– Exotic animals in particular may carry potential zoonotic infections.
– The patient may mistakenly understand the ESA to be an evidence-based treatment for depression and thus forego other treatments.
– Becoming certified as having a psychiatric disability carries many possible implications for the future, including: employment, professional licensing, security clearances, child custody disputes, ownership of firearms (in some localities), and other disability claims.

Perhaps this should go without saying, but the clinician who certifies an ESA should also be prepared to defend that determination in court in the event that this designation is ever challenged [12].

If you do agree to perform this evaluation, there is currently not a standard process for how it must be done. However, some experts have begun to map out guidelines, which you may find helpful. The assessment generally includes three components:

1. *Assessment of the patient*: What is the patient's diagnosis? Is the patient psychiatrically disabled? Is there a role for an ESA in the treatment plan?
2. *Assessment of the animal*: Is the animal capable of performing this clinical role? Keep in mind that not all animals are going to be cut out for this job. There has already been at least one (published) case of an emotional support animal requiring its own (second) emotional support animal on what must have been a very stressful plane flight [11].
3. *Observation of the interaction between the patient and the animal*: Can you demonstrate that the animal helps the patient to function when they are together?

If this strikes you as series of tasks that would be difficult to perform well from the primary care clinic, you may be right. But ultimately, the decision is up to you. Whatever you decide—in this and in any other interactions with the legal system, just be prepared to stand by it in court.

References

1. World Health Organization. Depression and other common mental disorders: global health estimates. Geneva: World Health Organization; 2017. License: CC BY-NC-SA 3.0 IGO
2. Mather L, Ropponen A, Mittendorfer-Rutz E, et al. Health, work and demographic factors associated with a lower risk of work disability and unemployment in employees with lower back, neck and shoulder pain. BMC Musculoskelet Disord. 2019;20:622.
3. Gaspar FW, Jolivet DN, Wizner K, et al. Pre-existing and new-onset depression and anxiety among workers with injury or illness work leaves. JOEM. 2020;62:e567–72.
4. Gaspar FW, Zaidel CS, Dewa CS. Rates and predictors of recurrent work disability due to common mental health disorders in the United States. PLoS One. 2018;13:e0205170.
5. Bass C, Wade DT. Malingering and factitious disorder. Pract Neurol. 2018:1–10.
6. Chisholm D, Sweeny K, Sheehan P, et al. Scaling-up treatment of depression and anxiety: a global return on investment analysis. Lancet Psychiatry. 2016;3:415–24.
7. Shuey KM, Wilson AE. Trajectories of work disability and economic insecurity approaching retirement. J Gerontol B Psychol Sci Soc Sci. 2019;74:1200–10.
8. Helgesson M, Tinghög P, Wang M, et al. Trajectories of work disability and unemployment among young adults with common mental disorders. BMC Public Health. 2018;18:1228.
9. Paunio T, Korhonen T, Hublin C, et al. Poor sleep predicts symptoms of depression and disability retirement due to depression. J Affect Disord. 2015;172:381–9.
10. Leinonen T, Solovieva S, Husgafvel-Pursiainen K, et al. Do individual and work-related factors differentiate work participation trajectories before and after vocational rehabilitation? PLoS One. 2019;14:e0212498.
11. Younggren JN, Boness CL, Bryant LM, Koocher GP. Emotional support animal assessments: toward a standard and comprehensive model for mental health professionals. Prof Psychol Res Pr. 2020;51:156–62.
12. American Psychological Association (APA). Emotional support animal position statement. https://www.apa-hai.org/resources/emotional-support-animal-position-statement/. Accessed 3/15/21 4:22pm.

Index

A

Abnormal Involuntary Movement Scale
  (AIMS), 67
Acute toxicity, 64
Adjunctive bupropion, 42
Adjustment disorder, 10
Antidepressant medications, 3
  activation and anxiety, 44
  best practices, 26–30
  bleeding, 39
  bupropion, 22
  convenience, 17
  costs, 17
  desired effects, 17
  diaphoresis, 45
  drug-drug interactions, 17
  effects on sleep, 43–44
  emotional detachment, 44
  expected side effects or risks, 17
  falls and fractures, 41
  gastrointestinal side effects, 43
  genetic testing, 18
  headaches, 44–45
  hepatotoxicity, 40
  hyponatremia, 40
  MAOIs, 25–26
  mirtazapine, 22
  QTc prolongation, 39–40
  seizures, 41
  serotonin syndrome, 38–39
  sexual dysfunction, 42–43
  SNRIs, 21–23
  SSRIs, 18–20
  suicidal ideation, 36, 37
  treatments, 30–31

tricyclic antidepressants, 23–25
vilazodone, 23
vortioxetine, 23
weight changes, 43
yawning, 45
Antipsychotic medications, 66–68
Anxiety disorder, 90
Ask Suicide Questionnaire (ASQ), 83
Ask Suicide-Screening Questions (ASQ)
  Toolkit, 84
Attention deficit/hyperactivity disorder
  (ADHD), 66
Atypical depression, 9
Augmentation, 63

B

Bipolar disorder, 1, 3, 11, 35
Bleeding, 39
Bupropion, 22, 41
Buspirone, 63

C

Chemical substances, 14
Cognitive behavioral therapy (CBT), 55–58
Columbia-Suicide Severity Rating Scale
  (C-SSRS), 83
C-SSRS Screener Version, 83–87
Cyclothymia, 11
Cytochrome P450 functioning, 18

D

Deep brain stimulation (DBS), 70

Printed in the United States
by Baker & Taylor Publisher Services